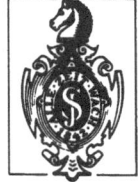

P. F. Schofield and E. W. Lupton (Eds.)

The Causation and Clinical Management of Pelvic Radiation Disease

Foreword by Dr. S. Goldberg

With 76 Figures

Springer-Verlag
London Berlin Heidelberg New York
Paris Tokyo Hong Kong

P. F. Schofield, MD, FRCS
Honorary Reader in Surgery, University of Manchester, Consultant
Surgeon, University Hospital of South Manchester, Manchester
M20 8LR UK

E. W. Lupton, MD, FRCS
Consultant Urologist, University Hospital of South Manchester,
Manchester M20 8LR UK

ISBN-13: 978-1-4471-1706-3   e-ISBN-13: 978-1-4471-1704-9

DOI: 10.1007/978-1-4471-1704-9

British Library Cataloguing in Publication Data
The causation and clinical management of pelvic radiation disease.
1. Man. Pelvic region. Diseases caused by radiotherapy
I. Schofield, P.F. (Philip F.), 1930–   II. Lupton, E.W. (Eric W.), 1946–
616.6'0642

Library of Congress Cataloging in Publication Data
The Causation and clinical management of pelvic radiation disease/edited by P.F.
Schofield and E.W. Lupton; foreword by S. Goldberg.
p. cm.
Includes bibliographies and index.

1. Pelvis—Cancer—Radiotherapy—Complications and sequelae. 2. Gastrointestinal
system—Radiation injuries. 3. Urinary organs—Radiation injuries. I.Schofield, P.F.
(Philip F.), 1930–   . II. Lupton, E.W. (Eric W.), 1946–
[DNLM: 1. Gastrointestinal Diseases—etiology. 2. Gastrointestinal Diseases—
therapy. 3. Radiotherapy—adverse effects. 4. Urogenital Neoplasms—radiotherapy.
5. Urologic Diseases—etiology. 6. Urologic Diseases—therapy. WI 100 C374]
RC280.P35C38   1989
616.3'3071—dc20
DNLM/DLC
for Library of Congress   89–11404 CIP

Softcover reprint of the hardcover 1st edition 1989

Filmset by Wilmaset, Birkenhead, Wirral

2128/3916–543210 (Printed on acid-free paper)

This book is dedicated to our wives,
Wendy and Joan

Foreword

It is now almost 100 years since Wilhelm Conrad Röntgen discovered X-rays in 1895. Today, radiation therapy has become a mainstay in the treatment of various pelvic malignancies. It is not surprising that a book devoted to this form of treatment and its accompanying complications should emanate from the largest cancer centre in the United Kingdom, the Christie Hospital. This book integrates into one volume the experience of distinguished surgeons and clinicians in dealing with the problems related to radiation in the pelvis.

The problems arising from this therapy can be very challenging requiring a multi-disciplined approach. This book brings together the experience of various disciplines and focuses on the management of the patient with major complications as well as minor ones.

Most of the contributors have been engaged in the study and treatment of pelvic malignancies for many years. What these authors have written not only expresses their own mature, individual opinions, but, taken as a whole, the book also provides a composite picture of the pathology and treatment of radiation injury as understood at the present time. In this volume, Drs. Schofield and Lupton have drawn on their vast clinical experience and set in perspective a modern approach to the care of the patient requiring pelvic radiation. Clinicians will be indebted for years to these authors for their efforts.

August, 1989   Stanley M. Goldberg, M.D., F.A.C.S.
                                          Clinical Professor of Surgery
                            Director, Division of Colon and Rectal Surgery
                                University of Minnesota Medical School
                                      Minneapolis, Minnesota, USA

Preface

It has been recognised for many years that radiation damage to the gastrointestinal and urinary tracts may occur as a complication of pelvic radiotherapy. During the early part of this decade there was an increase in radiation disease in several centres in the United Kingdom. The reasons for this sudden increase in bowel and urinary tract problems are complex. They include a change in the method of radiotherapy used in an attempt to improve the prognosis of carcinoma cervix by increasing the total radiation dose in some cases and the wider use of radiotherapy in other pelvic diseases.

The Christie Hospital is the largest cancer centre in the United Kingdom and treats, each year, approximately 400 new cases of carcinoma cervix, 400 new cases of carcinoma bladder and 200 new cases of carcinoma prostate. It is not surprising, therefore, that any increase in the complication rate will provide an expansion of the local coloproctological and urological involvement. The Manchester experience is, of course, not unique and over the years there is a considerable body of experience in the literature concerning radiation damage to the pelvic organs. The authors have drawn on the experience of other workers in this field to augment the knowledge gained from our concentrated exposure to a large number of cases. In the text we have attempted to assess other work in the field and to place it in context so that the book should be an internationally acceptable review of the present state of knowledge in this subject.

There has been a considerable surge of interest in radiation complications involving the urinary and gastrointestinal tracts in recent years. There are several reasons for this but probably the most significant has been the expansion of pelvic radiotherapy from the classical treatments of carcinoma cervix and bladder to include treatments for carcinoma prostate and carcinoma rectum. For this reason, many more clinicians have some experience of radiation disease. In the United States of America, it has been estimated that more than 50% of all patients with malignancy will have radiotherapy during the course of their management (Brady et al. 1985). Twenty-eight per cent of male malignancies are in either the prostate or bladder and almost 20% of female malignancy is in the uterus, ovary or bladder (American Cancer Society 1985). In both the USA and the UK many patients in these groups will receive radiotherapy. The above report indicates that in the USA about 40 000 new cases of carcinoma prostate per annum will receive radiation therapy and from the available evidence more than 10% will have some radiation-induced injury. An incidence of 11% of bowel injury is reported after pre-operative radiation and cystectomy for carcinoma bladder (Schellhammer et al. 1986). The incidence of serious complications after treatment for carcinoma of the cervix has been reported in many series and varies from 1% to 20% (Kjorstad et al. 1983).

The development of chemotherapy has led to protocols including this modality with radiotherapy and the combination has led to a higher incidence of radiation damage (Danjoux and Catton 1979).

It can be seen that these developments in treatment have led to an increased number of patients suffering from radiation-induced problems. Clearly there is a wide spectrum of radiation complications from the very minor to life-threatening disease. A system of grading of radiation complications was suggested by Pilepich and his colleagues in 1983 for patients with carcinoma prostate but it is useful for all patients with radiation-induced complications. The grading system is based on the effects on the patients' "performance status" and the necessity for therapy:

Grade I – minor symptoms which require no treatment.
Grade II – the symptoms do not affect the performance status and can be managed by simple outpatient methods.
Grade III – more severe symptoms altering the performance status. May have to be admitted for diagnostic procedures or minor surgery.
Grade IV – prolonged hospitalisation and major surgical intervention.
Grade V – fatal complications.

Most of this book relates to complications in grades III and IV though there is some mention of the lesser morbidity grades.

Part I of the book describes the principles and methods of radiotherapy for pelvic tumours and gives an historical account of their evolution. Pathology features, both macroscopic and microscopic, have been fascinating and, at times, bizarre. More large macroscopic specimens have been available from small and large bowel than from the urinary tract because more ablative surgery has been necessary in the gastrointestinal tract. Surgery on the urinary tract tended to be more reconstructive or diversionary. Radiological assessment of the bowel and urinary tract has yielded a most interesting collection of images, some of which represent extreme examples of features such as fistula or stricture development. It has sometimes been necessary to gain diagnostic accuracy and therapeutic assistance from new, more invasive procedures such as percutaneous catheterisation of the renal pelvis.

Parts II and III concentrate on clinical assessment and management. The problems encountered in both bowel and urinary tract are often challenging and difficult to manage. Some patients with extensive disease are very ill and the continuing morbidity and mortality rates are considerable in this group. One of the interesting features of radiation change is the time to development of symptoms and signs. It can take over 20 years for radiation sequelae to be declared. Emphasis must, therefore, be placed on the continued awareness of this potential diagnosis.

Our approach to these clinical problems has always been multidisciplinary so it was natural that when we turned to write about this subject we should use the same approach. We are grateful to our colleagues who have willingly contributed their expertise to the production of this book. It is hoped that at least some of our experience, imparted through this manuscript, will be of help to both surgical and non-surgical practitioners who deal only sporadically with pelvic radiation disease.

Philip F. Schofield
Eric W. Lupton

Manchester, 1989

References

Brady LW, Markoe AM, Sheline GE, Suntharalingham N, Sutherland RM (1985) Radiation oncology. Programs for the present and future. Cancer 55:2037–2050

Cancer facts and figures (1985) American Cancer Society, New York

Danjoux CE, Catton GE (1979) Delayed complications in colo-rectal carcinoma treated by combination radiotherapy and 5-fluorouracil. Eastern Cooperative Oncology Group: Pilot study. Int J Radiat Oncol Biol Phys 5:311–316

Kjorstad KE, Martimbeau PW, Iversen T (1983) Stage 1B carcinoma of the cervix, the Norwegian Radium Hospital: results and complications. Gynecol Oncol 15:42–47

Pilepich MV, Pajak T, George FW et al. (1983) Preliminary report on Phase III RTOG studies of extended-field irradiation in carcinoma of the prostate. Am J Clin Oncol (CCT) 6:485–491

Schellhammer PF, Jordan GH, El-Mahdi AM (1986) Pelvic complications after interstitial and external beam irradiation of urologic and gynaecologic malignancy. World J Surg 10:259–268

Acknowledgements

We wish to thank our nursing and junior medical colleagues for their considerable assistance in the care of patients with pelvic radiation disease. We acknowledge the significant clinical contribution of Mr. Robin Barnard to the management of urological problems. Our thanks are due to Dr Wendy Bellhouse, Mrs Gillian Trimble and Mrs Sharon Bracchi for typing the manuscript. We also wish to thank the Medical Illustration Department, University Hospital of South Manchester, and in particular Keith Harrison, for assistance with the illustrations. We are grateful to Michael Jackson, Medical Editor, Springer-Verlag, for his help and encouragement.

Contents

PART 2 BOWEL DISORDERS

PART 3 URINARY TRACT DISORDERS

7 Predisposing Factors, Clinical Features, Investigations: Radiation Urinary Tract Disease
E. W. Lupton

8 Treatment of Radiation Urinary Tract Disease
R. J. Barnard and E. W. Lupton

9 Conclusions and the Future
P. F. Schofield and E. W. Lupton

Contributors

R. J. Barnard, MB, FRCS
Consultant Urologist, University Hospital of South Manchester,
Manchester M20 8LR UK

N. D. Carr, MD, FRCS
Senior Registrar, St Mark's Hospital, City Road, London EC1V
2PS UK (formerly Research Fellow in Surgery, University Hospital
of South Manchester)

B. Eddleston, FRCR
Director of Diagnostic Radiology, Christie Hospital, Manchester
M20 9BX UK

N. Y. Haboubi, DPath, MRCPath, ChB
Consultant Histopathologist, University Hospital of South
Manchester, Manchester M20 8LR UK

P. S. Hasleton MD, MRCPath
Consultant Histopathologist, Wythenshawe Hospital, Manchester
M23 9LT UK

D. Holden, FRCS
Lecturer in Urology, University Hospital of South Manchester,
Manchester M20 8LR UK

R. D. Hunter, MD, FRCR
Director of Radiotherapy, Christie Hospital, Manchester M20 9BX
UK

R. J. Johnson, FRCR
Senior Lecturer, Department of Diagnostic Radiology, University
of Manchester, Honorary Consultant Radiologist, Christie Hospital,
Manchester M20 9BX UK

E. W. Lupton, MD, FRCS
Consultant Urologist, University Hospital of South Manchester,
Manchester M20 8LR UK

P. F. Schofield MD, FRCS
Honorary Reader in Surgery, University of Manchester, Consultant
Surgeon, University Hospital of South Manchester, Manchester
M20 8LR UK

P. M. Taylor, MB, ChB, MRCP, FRCR
Lecturer in Diagnostic Radiology, University of Manchester,
Manchester M13 9PT UK

Part 1
General Principles

1. Radiotherapy Techniques

R. Hunter

Introduction

Shortly after the discovery of radium in 1895, the event that marks the beginning of radiotherapy, malignant disease in the pelvis was treated with the new rays. Radium in a powder form was initially encapsulated in glass tubes. In that form it was placed in the uterus and vagina of patients with inoperable advanced malignant disease of the cervix. Within a decade, enthusiastic reports of high-grade palliation and long-term patient survival provoked great interest and radium became much more widely available. The early pioneers learnt to seal it into metal tubes or needles which filtered out unwanted poor quality radiation. They applied it safely to cavities and pushed it directly into the base of epithelial tumours. In this early form, radium came to be used in vesical, rectal, anal, urethral and even parametrial disease. Shortly after the recognition of the clinical efficacy came a realisation of the potentially harmful effects on the patients' normal tissues so that safe dosage systems for applying treatment to patients were formulated. Satisfactory radium systems were developed in the bigger European centres in Paris and Stockholm and modified into a very satisfactory inter-nationally usable form in Manchester (Tod 1947).

Radium's supremacy in the field of pelvic radiotherapy began to wane gradually as higher energy x-ray machines became available during the 1930s but, until the development of the linear accelerator and the telecobalt unit immediately after the end of the second world war, it remained the mainstay of any pelvic radiotherapy treatment. The modern computerised, electronically controlled linear accelerators can satisfactorily irradiate tumours of any size homogeneously no matter what their site in the pelvis, with techniques that are relatively simple to reproduce and reliable in their execution. The development of higher energy linear accelerators greatly simplified the radiotherapy of pelvic malignant disease and, for a number of years, radium techniques became less commonly used. In the last decade after the development of satisfactory artificial radionuclides and a more critical reappraisal of the success of, and complications associated with, the x-ray techniques, there has been a revival of interest in modern techniques based on the radium system (Cole and Hunter 1985).

The modern radiotherapist has a variety of satisfactory techniques to treat patients with pelvic malignant disease. The most commonly used is teletherapy in which beams of ionising radiation from a megavoltage source, a linear accelerator or a telecobalt machine, are directed onto the target volume while the patient lies alone in a fully shielded treatment room. An essential part of gynaecological radiotherapy is intracavitary therapy where artificial radionuclides sealed in a carrier material are placed temporarily in the cavities of the uterus and vagina. The least used technique is interstitial therapy in which a radioactive material contained in a "carrier" is placed temporarily or permanently in the tumour and its immediately surrounding tissues. Occasionally, radionuclides in colloid form have been injected permanently into tissues such as the prostate.

The radiations used in most of the standard techniques are γ rays and x-rays. X-rays are produced by a machine and γ rays are the products of a radionuclide but physically they are identical. The radiation is in the form of photons (or packets of energy) with a capacity to penetrate tissues. The penetrating power depends on the quality of the beam and is usually expressed as kilovoltage or megavoltage. The higher the energy the greater the penetrating power. In clinical radiotherapy of pelvic malignant disease, megavoltage beams from linear accelerators with energies of 4–25 meV are preferred because they do not produce significant skin reactions on flat surfaces, penetrate deeply into the biggest pelvis and are not significantly affected by passage through the pelvic bones.

All radiotherapy techniques produce their effect at a clinical level in exactly the same way. The photons of the x-ray machines and the γ rays of the telecobalt and radionuclides ionise the chemical structure of cells. From a practical point of view, the process is instantaneous but the damage to the fine molecular structure of the tumour and normal tissue may take days, weeks or years to manifest itself. The pattern of ionisation is a random process within the cell but the deoxyribonucleic acid (DNA) of the nucleus is particularly sensitive to any damage and critically so at the time of cell division. Any ionising radiation entering tissue starts to deposit energy in the cells through which it passes and, by a variety of physical processes, this damages the fine chemical structures of the different intracellular molecules. The net effect is that the energy of the beam is lost steadily as it passes into the patient and permanent intracellular damage results. There is nothing to suggest that, at this cellular level, malignant cells are different from normal tissue cells in their response to radiation. The sensitivity of human cells to ionising radiation depends on their physical state, the current phase of the cell cycle, their environment and particularly the adequacy of cellular oxygenation.

Clinical radiotherapy developed empirically and it is only in recent years that the scientific study of the interaction of ionising radiation with cells and tissues has explained the phenomena that have been observed in clinical practice (Hall 1988).

Malignant tumours, even when small and localised, are now recognised to have a heterogeneous population of cells; some are part of the malignant population while others are derived from the surrounding normal healthy tissue. Among the malignant cells are a group, usually small, which are the true heart of the disease. These cells are capable of infinite cell division in the correct environment. At any one time, most of the malignant cells are actively dividing but a small number are recognised to be resting. Mixed with the malignant cells are normal blood vessels, connective tissue cells and leucocytes.

Most malignant human tumours are now believed to develop from a single abnormal cell (monoclonal) but the disease that we see, feel and treat contains a minimum of 10^8 malignant cells and often 10^{10} cells. Recognisable disease is the product of at least 36 cell divisions. Since the complete cell cycle of a human tumour cell can take anything from a few days to a few months, the natural history of human pelvic malignant tumours is long and may be a number of years. It is only in the last part of this time that the tumour is clinically apparent.

The majority of malignant cells visible histologically in a human tumour are not of prime importance because many are incapable of continued infinite cell division, some are shed from surfaces and others are dying naturally. An important reason for this last phenomenon is that tumour growth is accompanied by a new blood supply from the surrounding normal tissue. This is carried by thin-walled, poorly organised vessels with sluggish flow which leads to infarction and haemorrhage. As a result, the centre of most tumour nodules is poorly supplied with oxygen and nutrients, a situation which has been found to make them relatively resistant to ionising radiation. Prior to radiotherapy any tumour can be considered as a poorly organised heterogeneous mixture of cells at different stages of development.

Ionising radiation works by a random process of damage to the cells of the tumour. The critical damage to the DNA of the nucleus is only expressed at the time of cell division by the death of the cell. Similar damage of a random nature may occur to normal cells supporting the area of disease and to any adjacent tissue which is included in the treatment field.

Within the true pelvis there are a number of tissues which react differently to radiotherapy. The bladder, uterus, vagina, rectum and small bowel all have a similar structure: an epithelial layer, a supporting stroma, a muscle layer and blood vessels with an endothelial and smooth muscle component. To understand what happens after therapeutic radiation it is helpful to consider each dividing cell group as a different population with its own balance of dividing to resting cells. Radiation damage to all these cells takes place at the instant the patient is treated but the effects of that damage take differing times to appear in the different cell populations. A certain percentage of the dividing cells in each group will sustain permanent damage. The extent of this will depend on the dose delivered. For the columnar cells of the rectum this means that within 5 to 7 days there will be a failure to produce new cells to replace the cells that are being constantly and naturally shed from the surface. If this process is severe enough there will be visible changes with fibrin formation on the rectal mucosa at 7–10 days. The changes persist until the basal layer cells that have escaped lethal injury repopulate the crypts and the epithelium.

In the bladder the much slower turnover rate of the epithelial stem cells makes symptomatic acute reactions slower to appear and, normally, less significant. Little will be seen on cystoscopic examination at this time.

The cervical and vaginal mucosa, which in intracavitary therapy are subjected to very high local doses, will show a fibrinous reaction at 7–10 days after treatment. In the absence of local infection the patient has a minor serous discharge but little else in the way of symptoms.

Amongst all the different cell populations, the stromal and vascular endothelial cells in any of the pelvic organs respond most slowly as they have long natural cell kinetics. These vascular and connective tissue changes are the basis of the significant injuries of "late" radiation disease. This process which takes place to some extent in all therapeutically irradiated tissues, can lead to ischaemia, infarction and necrosis and is discussed more fully in Chapter 2. On the other hand, the normal reserves within human tissues may allow them to look relatively normal macroscopically after good quality radical radiotherapy yet subtle changes exist which may become manifest later, particularly after subsequent surgery (Galland and Spencer 1986). Like the acute reactions, these late responses are dose dependent, but there seems little association between the protracted acute and serious late complications. Acute reactions can be lessened or avoided by increasing the number of fractions and overall treatment time but late complications are only modified by lowering the effective dose.

Using modern equipment for planning of homogeneous treatment volumes and careful intracavitary and interstitial techniques, radiation morbidity can be controlled but it cannot be eliminated. Tolerance limits for all treatments are well established. Treatments are based on daily fractions, which are continued for 5 days per week for a number of weeks. In planning any treatment, the problem that faces the radiotherapist is that as the primary tumour size increases, the dose required to "sterilise" the tumour increases which, in turn, increases the risk to the normal supporting and surrounding tissues. The majority of primary carcinomas which are in the pelvis are only moderately sensitive to ionising radiation and in practice it becomes necessary to balance cancer control against morbidity. The final choice of dose for any particular treatment often depends on the morbidity level that is acceptable. A second problem is that the relationship between cancer control or radiation injury and dose is not a linear one. Dose–response relationships of this type are thought to be better represented by sigmoid curves so that small changes in final biological dose can produce very significant changes in both control and morbidity. If the two curves are close together then increased control may only be realised by a major increase in morbidity (Fig. 1.1).

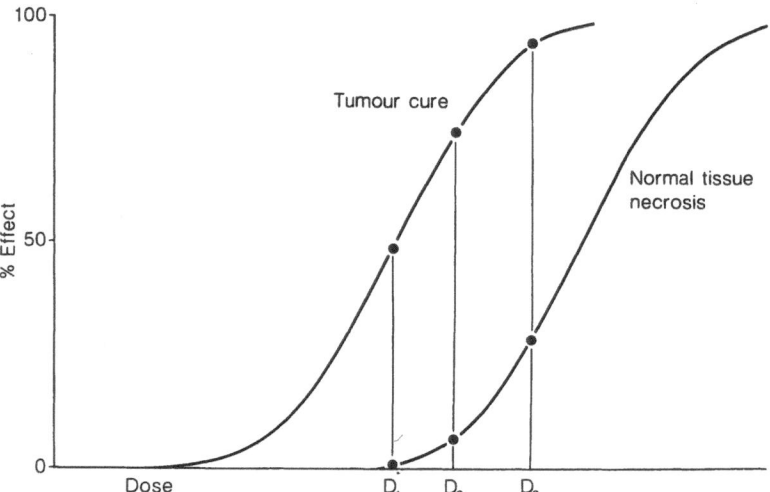

Fig. 1.1. Diagrammatic representation of sigmoid dose–response curves for cancer control and morbidity showing three possible radiation doses: D1 poor control, no morbidity; D2 reasonable control with small level of morbidity; D3 maximum control but unacceptable morbidity.

Radiation damage to normal tissue is inevitable in clinical radiotherapy and may result in a spectrum of late tissue effects from very mild asymptomatic changes of one organ function to major life-threatening incidents involving more than one tissue. The position of the different organs relative to each other and the tumour dominates the response to treatment. In any pelvic treatment this results in multiple tissues being irradiated and, therefore, exposed to potential side effects.

To understand the types of radiation injury which may occur we must now consider techniques used in the treatment of the major pelvic tumours in more detail.

Carcinoma Bladder

The aim of the initial assessment is to identify the tumour position and volume with the patient in the supine position. Cystoscopic assessment of the individual patient remains the best investigative procedure because the site, size and stage of the primary disease can be defined and accurate histology can be obtained by biopsy. It is also important to assess the rest of the bladder and urethra for additional foci of urothelial malignancy or other abnormality. The size and nature of the prostate may be relevant. A cystogram is subsequently performed with a limited amount of contrast solution and appropriate films are taken with markers applied to the skin surfaces. The information from the cystogram is then combined with that from intravenous urogram (IVU), cystoscopy and examination under anaesthesia (EUA) to estimate the site and size of the disease in order to define a treatment plan. Ultrasonography and computerised tomographic (CT) scanning are useful ancillary tools to define the tumour volume, the degree of infiltration and, sometimes, the presence of enlarged pelvic nodes (Rose and Shipley 1988). CT scanning in the treatment position is often combined with the previous investigations to improve the accuracy of planning (Fig. 1.2). This is particularly useful in large or fundal tumours because conventional planning systems have been shown to be inaccurate.

There are several techniques for treating bladder tumours and a final decision may depend upon the size of the patient and the site of the disease. Carcinoma bladder is such a common radiotherapeutic problem that simple rotation or multiple field isocentric techniques are normally used (Fig. 1.3). Some radiotherapists concentrate entirely on the defined tumour volume while others start treating the whole true pelvis and cone down on the defined volume towards the end of the treatment. There is no real evidence that either technique gives better results.

The radical x-ray therapy of bladder carcinoma is a punishing treatment and is difficult to accomplish satisfactorily as an outpatient. Before the radiotherapy, bladder infections should be treated and any outlet obstruction relieved by transurethral resection. Haematuria, even if heavy, usually stops after 1–2 weeks of active radiotherapy.

An acute bowel and bladder reaction is inevitable with radical radiotherapy. The bladder reaction produces a predictable increase in frequency, aggravating what may be a troublesome symptom already. The severity of bowel symptoms is

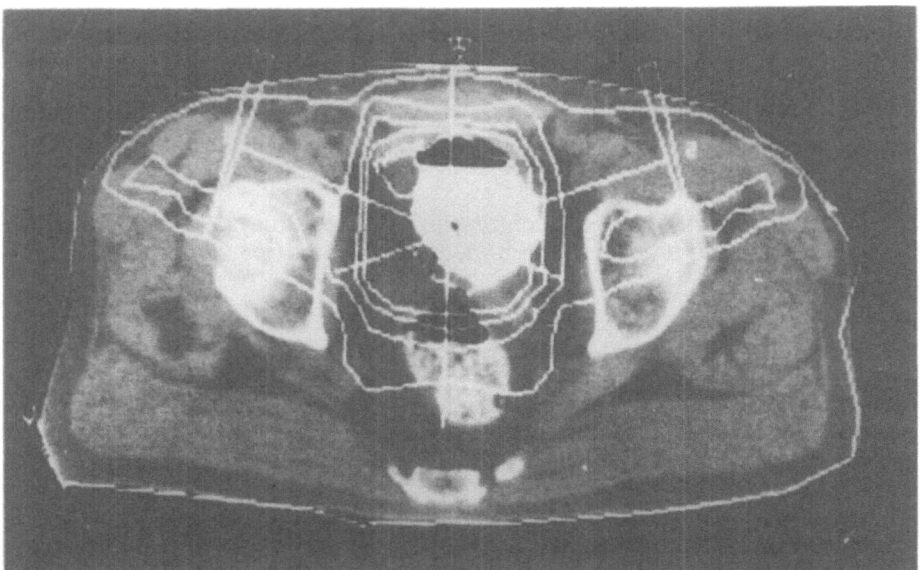

Fig. 1.2. CT scan of the pelvis of patient with carcinoma bladder. The radiation beams are simulated and the central volume receiving the planned dose is outlined. This includes the tumour, normal bladder and some surrounding normal tissue.

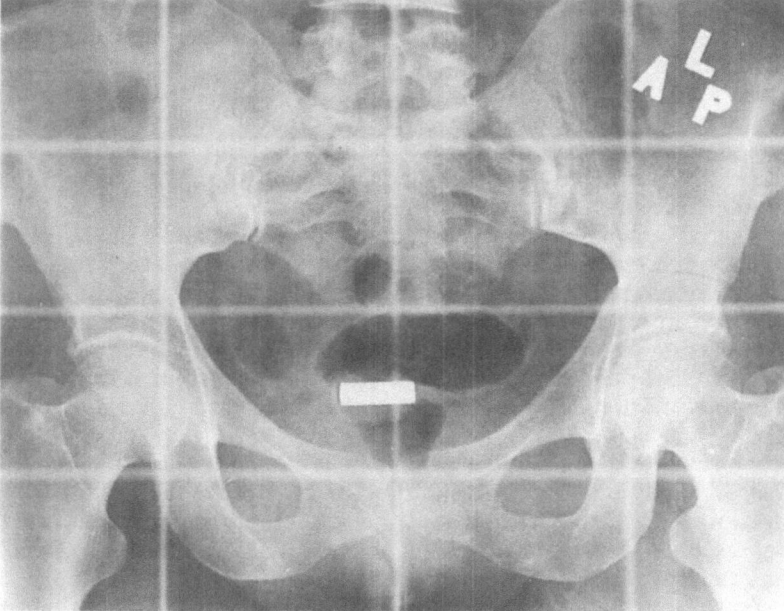

Fig. 1.3. Antero-posterior radiograph of pelvis of patient receiving a typical external beam treatment. The radiation field is contained within the central rectangle outlined by the wires.

unpredictable. In women, the uterus may help to keep the small bowel away from the bladder. In men, small bowel loops and sigmoid colon are inevitably within the high-dose treatment volume for fundal tumours and the rectum is in the high-dose volume for basal tumours. Significant doses of radiation are received by some part of the bowel in all patients, leaving damage which manifests itself as an acute reaction.

Palliative treatments tend to be much simpler in planning and execution with low doses being delivered to large volumes of the pelvis. Case selection for palliative treatment is aimed at identifying patients who will live long enough to benefit from control of haematuria but may not live long enough to develop complications. Inevitably some of them do.

Carcinoma Prostate

Fifteen years ago, there was little radiotherapeutic interest in the treatment of carcinoma of the prostate. The disease was considered to be a poorly responsive adenocarcinoma situated awkwardly around the urethra and the base of the bladder. More recently, clinical studies have established that primary tumour control can be achieved with radical radiotherapy of small primary tumours (Ray and Bagshaw, 1975; Jazy et al. 1979). In spite of this the place of radiotherapy remains controversial because of the long natural history of the disease in many patients, the alternative techniques for primary control and the advanced age of many patients. Most radiotherapists will now accept for radical radiotherapy patients with primary disease confined to a prostate of normal size or with moderate enlargement. We prefer to restrict active treatment to patients below 70 years of age whose general condition is good.

In most centres, radical radiotherapy involves the use of megavoltage teletherapy techniques very similar to those employed in carcinoma of the bladder but normally using a high dose to a smaller volume of tissue. Assessment of the volume for treatment is aided by EUA and cystoscopy, ultrasonography and CT scanning. In this type of treatment the margin around the defined tumour includes the base of the bladder and the anterior rectal wall. An acute proctitis is inevitable after this course of treatment. The radiation tolerance of these tissues low in the pelvis is recognised to be less than that of the perivesical tissues and a 10% reduction in biological dose relative to a similar bladder treatment is commonly employed.

A small number of radiotherapeutic enthusiasts continue to promote interstitial techniques in which permanent ^{125}I seeds or temporary implants of ^{192}Ir wire are placed carefully into the prostatic tumour at open operation in collaboration with a urologist. These techniques allow reactions to be confined to the diseased tissue and can restrict the dangers of late tissue complications but this advantage has to be balanced against the need for open surgery and the hazards of handling and implanting radioactive materials. A potentially safer and more accurate method of interstitial radiotherapy is transperineal ^{125}I seed implantation guided by transrectal ultrasonography and performed under epidural anaesthesia (Holm et al. 1983).

Carcinoma Cervix

The radical treatment of carcinoma of the cervix by radiotherapy has evolved over the last 80 years. Initially, intracavitary therapy was the only treatment but with machine developments teletherapy has become an integral part of treatment. It would be unusual for a centre not to use both techniques. However, the balance between the contribution of the two techniques to the total dose can vary widely between patients with different stages of the disease and between different radiotherapy centres.

The teletherapy part of the treatment is often given first and is the easier to accomplish. Using high energy linear accelerators satisfactory homogeneous treatments can be given to the true pelvis or an extended pelvic field or even to the pelvis and para-aortic region. Most frequently the treatment is confined to the true pelvis and, to spare some unnecessary bowel irradiation, this is accomplished by the use of a second pair of lateral fields. These are colloquially known as "box techniques" (Fig. 1.4). The final decision about the volume to be irradiated can depend upon information obtained by clinical examination under anaesthesia, intravenous pyelogram (IVP), ultrasonography and, in some centres, lymphangiography and CT scanning (Brady et al. 1987).

External beam therapy is normally given daily, 5 days per week for 3 to 5 weeks and during this time there is often some regression of the bulkier primary tumours. This helps to restore the normal anatomy and makes optimal positioning of the intracavitary sources easier.

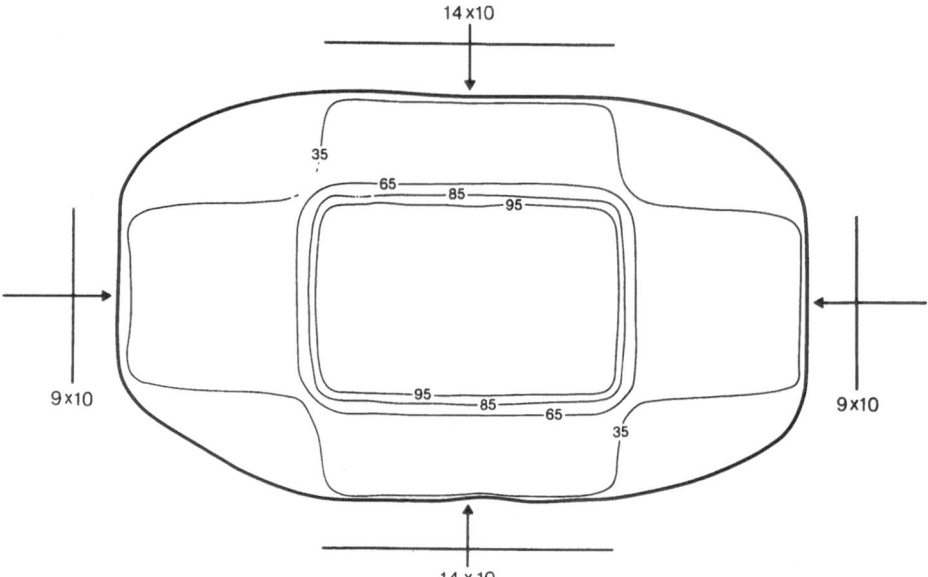

Fig. 1.4. Diagram of the transverse section of the pelvis of a patient being treated by a box technique. Only the volume in the central area enclosed by the four beams receives the full prescribed dose.

At the end of their teletherapy the patients have an acute pelvic radiation reaction with its associated bowel irritability and urinary frequency. This must be sufficiently settled to allow the patient to be confined to bed for up to 3 days during the planned intracavitary therapy.

There are a variety of intracavitary techniques depending on the experience of the radiotherapist, the equipment available and the needs of the individual patient. In all of them the direction and length of the uterus is determined by a sound. The cervix is dilated to allow the passage of a tube of approximately 8 mm in diameter into the body of the uterus. This is either allowed to extend down into the vagina until it is distal to the tumour or separate tubes are placed in the upper vaginal lateral fornices (Fig. 1.5). These are retained in position either by gauze packing, by the vaginal applicator or by a stitch at the introitus.

Originally, uterine and vaginal applicators were made of cork or rubber and the radioactive material was radium. More recently, they have been manufactured of

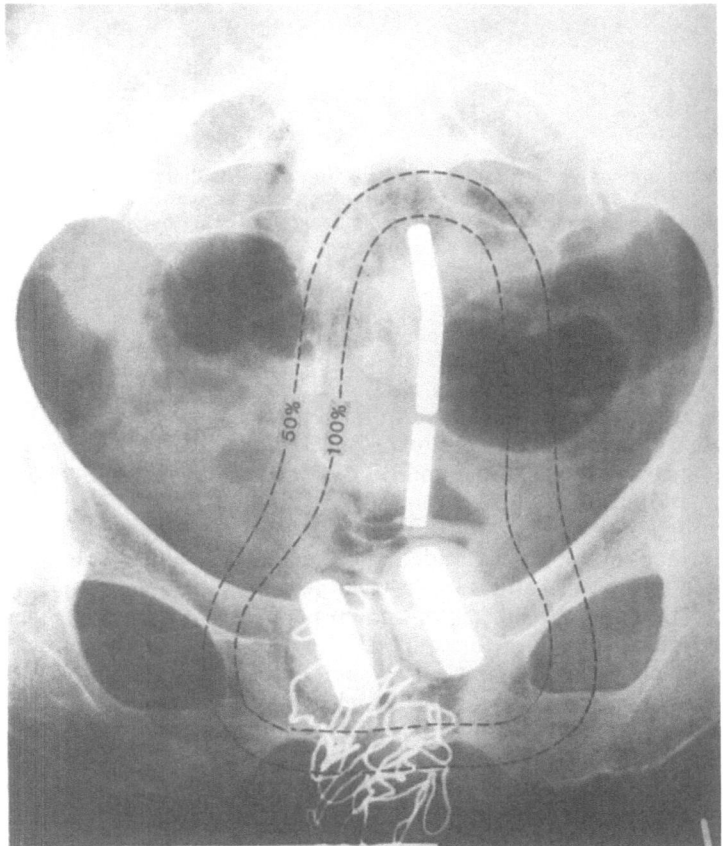

Fig. 1.5. Antero-posterior radiograph of the pelvis of a patient having intracavitary therapy for carcinoma of the cervix using classical Manchester preloaded applicators. The isodose distribution is represented by the pear-shaped lines around the applicator. The steep dose gradients in this treatment mean that the outer line receives half of the dose of the inner line.

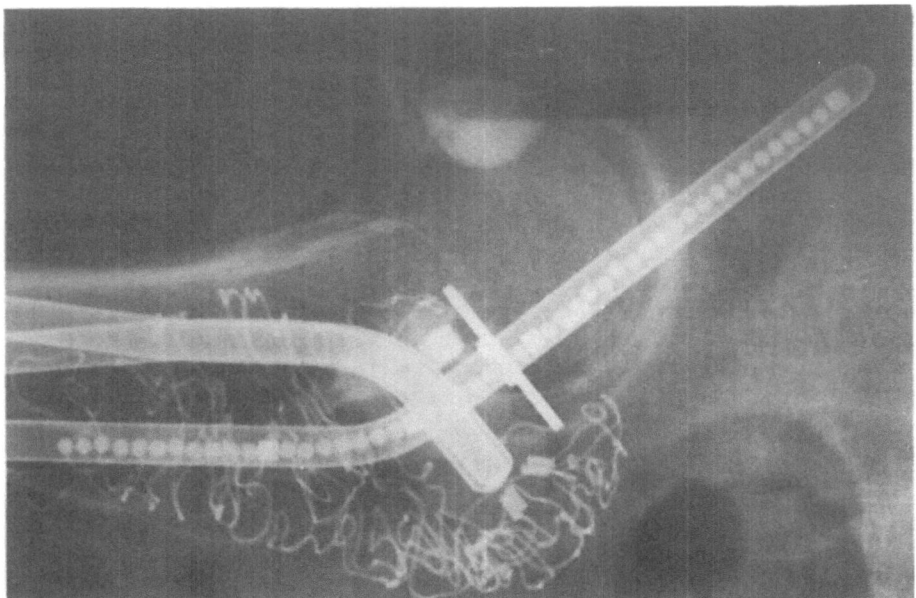

Fig. 1.6. Lateral radiograph of pelvis of patient having intracavitary therapy using modern afterloading applicators. This demonstrates the proximity of adjacent normal tissues. The Foley catheter is drawn down to the base of the bladder which contains air. The air bubble in the recto-sigmoid lies postero-lateral to the posterior fornix and gauze packing separates the applicator from the vaginal mucosa and rectum.

plastic or light steels and radium has been replaced by artificial radionuclides such as caesium (^{137}Cs) and cobalt (^{60}Co).

Intracavitary therapy may be completed in a single session or delivered in a number of separate treatments over a period of 2 or 3 weeks. The choice depends on the stage of the disease, the general condition of the patient, the dosage given by the external beam therapy and the equipment available.

Using modern techniques to avoid staff exposure to ionising radiation in operating areas, the active sources are loaded into the hollow applicators after the patient has returned to the ward and is in her treatment position (Fig. 1.6). If the sources are loaded by hand the system is known as manual afterloading. The more sophisticated techniques allow the sources to be loaded by remote control in a radiologically protected environment (O'Connell et al. 1965). There are now satisfactory radionuclide sources available which deliver the planned dose in minutes, hours or days resulting in a high, medium or low dose rate, respectively (Cole and Hunter 1985).

Much clinical research work has been done to evolve satisfactory regimes using these approaches. At one extreme there are low-dose techniques in which the treatment mirrors the 3–6 days continuous treatment of the classical radium systems. Treatment is normally in one or two sessions and the doses are those established from the days of radium. Over the last two decades there have been moves to decrease the treatment time to a matter of hours or minutes. These changes of dose rate result in changes of biological effect and mean that the absolute dose given may have to be reduced or the number of sessions increased. When these different low, medium and high dose rate systems are used optimally there is probably little to choose between them in terms of cancer control or morbidity.

Intracavitary therapy is a very important potential source of localised radiation injury to all the central pelvic tissues. Although the sources are mounted in applicators, the radiation dose on the surface of the applicators is high. As the radiation spreads out into the pelvis the dose falls quickly. The distribution of radiation dosage is designed to treat adequately the carcinoma of the cervix but in the course of accomplishing this the other organs in the pelvis are irradiated to some degree. An important factor influencing this is the internal anatomy of the individual patient's pelvis. For example, if the standard applicators of the Manchester system are correctly placed in the upper vagina, the bladder may or may not be an anterior relation of the radiation sources. Similar situations arise with the rectum, sigmoid colon and small bowel throughout the three-dimensional pelvic treatment. Many factors including the thickness and position of the uterus, the length and capacity of the vagina, the bulk of the tumour, the size and shape of the bladder and the length and position of the sigmoid colon contribute to the final pattern of exposure of the normal tissues. Exposure of the lower rectum and anal canal is the most predictable and easiest to control. Normally, some sort of packing or shielding is placed between the upper vaginal applicators and the posterior vaginal wall. Unless the vault is small, this is enough to avoid injury from the intracavitary therapy. Many centres make a direct reading of the rectal dose by placing an ionisation chamber temporarily in the rectum at the end of the insertion procedure and estimating the dose rate to the anterior rectal wall (Bourne et al. 1983; Cole and Hunter 1985). Others put a radio-opaque marker in the rectum to allow a calculation of the dose rate to rectal points, usually on the anterior wall.

The dose to the empty or drained bladder depends mainly on mural thickness, capacity and the length of the vagina. CT investigations of patients undergoing treatment have revealed how variable the position and shape of the bladder can be during identical treatments in different patients. When patients are receiving the same prescribed dose, the maximum bladder dosage can vary from 50%–130% of the presumed value. If, instead of placing the sources in the upper vagina they are extended down towards the introitus, the dose to the bladder base and urethra will rise considerably. This can be calculated by utilising a radio-opaque urinary catheter and opacifying the balloon. It is much more difficult and unusual to make any attempt to calculate ureteric dosage and it is fortunate that the ureters are less commonly the site of damage.

For the small bowel and sigmoid colon the uterine sources are the potential cause of damage. Probably the most significant factor influencing this is the thickness of the uterus. Patients with a small diameter uterus or an asymmetrical cavity may inadvertently receive a high bowel dosage during an apparently normal treatment schedule. Anything that reduces normal bowel motility, intra-abdominal adhesions, pelvic inflammatory disease or anaesthesia will tend to exacerbate this problem. Clinical experience suggests that sources placed in a retroverted or a long uterus more easily injure bowel than those in the normal anteverted midline uterus. Most intracavitary therapy planning does not take into account these variables, which are usually unknown. As a result, there is a poor correlation between dosage and central pelvic morbidity.

Carcinoma Rectum

The place of radiotherapy in the management of invasive carcinoma of the rectum remains uncertain. Paterson (1948) listed adenocarcinoma of the rectum as a radioresistant disease. However, significant papers have been published demonstrating that localised carcinoma can be cured and recurrent disease controlled by radiotherapy. This apparent conflict is resolved when the problem of irradiating the disease is considered.

Accurate definition of tumour volume has always been difficult except in very small and very low tumours. Even modern CT scanning techniques do not discriminate well between malignant and normal tissue in the posterior pelvis. Endorectal ultrasound has recently been suggested to give better definition (Benyon et al. 1986). If the volume is poorly defined, it is necessary to allow an increased field size, which inevitably involves increasing the volume of normal bowel irradiated. In addition, except in the most unusual situation, the full circumference of the rectum over a significant length has to be included in the treatment. Fear of significant bowel reaction dictates a dose of radiation 10%–20% less than that suitable for an equivalent-sized carcinoma of the bladder. The reduced chance of cancer control in the rectum by radiotherapy is because of this lower dosage of tolerable treatment rather than the fact that the tumour is an adenocarcinoma. This restricts curative radiotherapy to small tumours and patients unfit for surgery. In some centres these patients with low-lying, solitary, small tumours have, for many years, been offered local intracavitary radiotherapy either through an endoscope or by interstitial implantation (Papillon 1975). These techniques, if successful, can result in excellent control with sphincter retention and very localised normal tissue effects. Selection has to be by a joint agreement with a surgeon and careful follow up is mandatory. This approach is only suitable for less than 10% of patients with rectal cancer (Schofield and James 1983). The advantage for the patient is that the procedure is completed quickly and results in a very localised radiation reaction. There will be an acute proctitis and some danger of late necrosis but uninvolved tissues of the pelvis are not significantly irradiated and are at no real risk of injury.

Most rectal carcinomas have spread outside the rectal wall and about 10% are totally fixed to surrounding structures. For the carcinoma with moderate extrarectal spread it is still uncertain whether pre-operative or post-operative adjuvant radiotherapy is useful. Pre-operative radiotherapy has been given in subtolerance doses followed by immediate surgery. There is little reaction and there has been no adverse effect on the subsequent surgery (Cummings 1986).

Although it could certainly be argued that prospective adjuvant trials in selected patients may yet reveal significant benefits, the present opinion is that pre-operative radiotherapy improves pelvic control but does not influence survival (Jones et al. 1988). If the tumour is fixed, the method of choice is to give high-dose radiation within tolerance limits and allow 6–8 weeks for tumour regression before surgery (James and Schofield 1985). Some regression usually occurs and occasionally there is no identifiable tumour at surgery. At the dosage employed, transient bowel upset occurs but late radiation disease has been rare.

Immediate post-operative radiotherapy after surgery for carcinoma rectum carries more risk of both early and late radiation disease. In this situation, the small bowel is at particular risk (Romsdahl and Withers 1978). A difficult and regular problem remains that of the patient with local pelvic recurrence who is troubled by rectal mucous discharge with or without bleeding or perineal pain. There is no doubt that simple palliative beam radiotherapy based on a two field wedge or rotation techniques, with the patient lying prone, can improve symptoms for several months if the problem comes from the pelvis and not from more widespread disease (Schofield and James 1983).

The planning, dosage and fractionation should be aimed at avoiding unnecessary acute bowel reactions but in the post-operative pelvis, particularly after abdomino–perineal resection, loops of large or small bowel may be attached by benign or malignant adhesions so that no amount of care in planning, including the use of CT scanning will avoid "unnecessary" radiation being delivered to these tissues. In consequence, the radiotherapist has to treat a large volume of the posterior pelvis and balance the degree of palliation against the disability of the acute small or large bowel reactions which result. Few patients treated for local recurrence will live long enough to get late radiation damage.

References

Benyon J, Mortensen NJMcC, Foy DMA, Channer JL, Virjee J, Goddard P (1986) Pre-operative assessment of local invasion in rectal cancer: digital examination, endoluminal sonography or computed tomography? Br J Surg 73:1015–1017

Bourne RG, Kearsley JH, Grove WD, Roberts SJ (1983) The relationship between early and late gastrointestinal complications of radiation therapy for carcinoma of the cervix. Int J Radiat Oncol Biol Phys 9:1445–1450

Brady LW, Markoe AM, Micaily B, Dansker JI, Karlsson VL, Amendola BE (1987) Clinical treatment planning in gynaecologic cancer. Front Radiat Oncol 21:302–332

Cole MP, Hunter RD (1985) Female genital tract. In: Easson EC, Pointon RCS (eds) The radiotherapy of malignant disease. Springer, Berlin Heidelberg New York, pp 280–309

Cummings BJ (1986) A critical review of adjuvant pre-operative radiation therapy for adenocarcinoma of the rectum. Br J Surg 75:332–338

Galland RB, Spencer J (1986) The surgical management of radiation enteritis. Surgery 99:133–138

Hall EJ (1988) Radiobiology for the radiologist, 3rd edn. JB Lippincott & Co, Philadelphia

Holm HH, Juul N, Pedersen JF, Hansen H, Stroyer I (1983) Transperineal ^{125}I seed implantation in prostatic cancer guided by transrectal ultrasonography. J Urol 130:283–286

James RD, Schofield PF (1985) Resection of "inoperable" rectal cancer following radiotherapy. Br J Surg 72:279–281

Jazy FK, Aron B, Dettmer CM, Shehata WM (1979) Radiation therapy as definitive treatment for localised carcinoma of prostate. Urology 14:555–560

Jones DJ, Zaloudik J, James RD, Moore M, Schofield PF (1988) Local recurrence after pre-operative radiotherapy and surgery in rectal cancer. Br J Surg 75:1244

O'Connell D, Howard N, Joslin CA, Ramsey NW, Liversage WE (1965) A new remotely controlled unit for the treatment of uterine cancer Lancet ii:570–571

Papillon J (1975) Intracavity irradiation of early rectal cancer for cure: a review of 186 cases. Cancer 36:696

Paterson JRK (1948) The treatment of malignant disease by radium and x-rays: being a practice of radiotherapy. Edward Arnold & Co, London

Ray GR, Bagshaw MA (1975) The role of radiation therapy in the definitive treatment of adenocarcinoma of the prostate. Ann Rev Med 26:567–588

Romsdahl MM, Withers HR (1978) Radiotherapy combined with curative surgery. Its use as therapy for carcinoma of the sigmoid colon and rectum. Ann Surg 113:446–453

Rose MA, Shipley WU (1988) Radiation therapy in invasive bladder cancer: principles, results, patient selection and innovations. In: Raghavan D (ed) The management of bladder cancer. Edward Arnold & Co, London, pp 154–173

Schofield PF, James RD (1983) Treatment of carcinoma rectum and anus. In: Irving MH, Beart R (eds) International medical reviews, surgery 3, gastroenterological surgery. Butterworths, London, pp 198–217
Tod MC (1947) Optimum dosage in the treatment of cancer of the cervix by radiation. Acta Radiol 28:564–575

Suggested Further Reading

Hall EJ (1988) Radiobiology for the radiologist, 3rd edn. JB Lippincott & Co, Philadelphia
Easson EC, Pointon RCS (eds) (1985) The radiotherapy of malignant disease. Springer, Berlin Heidelberg New York
Raghaven D (ed) (1988) The management of bladder cancer. Edward Arnold & Co, London

2. Pathology of Radiation Injury

N. Y. Haboubi and P. S. Hasleton

"When treating tumours with high radiosensitivity in tissues of relatively low radiosensitivity, few complications of therapy occur."

Morgan Berthrong (1986)

Introduction

Irradiation is widely used in the treatment of some malignant tumours. It has become the therapy of choice in certain circumstances where surgery and/or chemotherapy have failed to produce good results. With increasing use, we have become more aware of the complications and potential hazards of radiotherapy. This chapter aims to describe the pathological changes after radiation to the bowel and the urogenital tracts. Both systems are affected due to their inclusion in the pelvic irradiation field. The commonest pelvic tumour requiring radiotherapy arises within the uterine cervix but tumours of the uterine body, ovaries, vagina, bladder, prostate and rectum are being increasingly treated by radiotherapy.

To understand radiation-induced injury it is important to comprehend the biological response of cells to radiation. During division cells replicate their chromatin in the S and G2 phases. Usually the cells are at their peak of radiosensitivity at the points of S and G2 of the cell cycle (Fig. 2.1). As cells with high turnover go more often through phases S and G2 in a given time than those

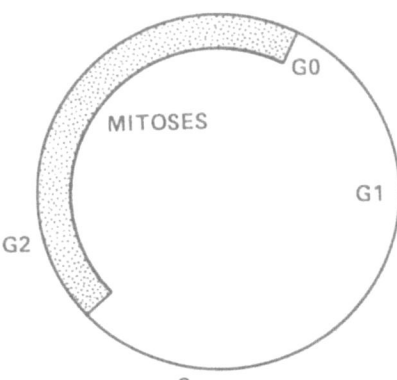

Fig. 2.1. A diagram to illustrate the cell cycle. The time of highest vulnerability of the cell is during mitosis and the G2 phase.

with low turnover, it follows that cells that divide more rapidly, such as the epithelial lining cells of the gut, are more prone to show radiation damage soon after radiotherapy. Conversely, cells with a lower rate of turnover like the endothelial cells and fibroblasts will show damage later.

The epithelial cells which have a high turnover rate and are affected more at the early stage of the disease, have the capacity for rapid regeneration and may resume a total or almost total cell population after a few weeks of injury. Following the recovery of the epithelial cells, the fibrovascular tissue starts to manifest pathological changes. It is common to see relatively normal mucosa with severely fibrotic and vascularly compromised subjacent tissue in late radiation disease.

The differential of sensitivity to radiation between the neoplasm and the adjacent exposed normal tissue is small, thus it must be expected that there will be radiation injury to some normal tissues (Berthrong 1986). The bowel and urinary tracts are at particular risk in radiotherapy directed to the pelvis. Interested pathologists have begun to gain wide experience in this field but this experience is largely confined to late disease. Although acute radiation injury is a common problem it is transient and rarely requires surgical intervention (Schofield 1987). Late radiation bowel disease produces irreversible complications which more often affect large areas of the gut and the urinary system. These result in surgical intervention which generates material for pathological assessment. Lack of biopsies in the early disease makes it difficult to study the evolution of this phase in humans.

Generally there is no single pathognomonic histological marker of late radiation bowel disease (Fajardo 1982). A combination of histological features enables the pathologist to suggest irradiation injury. In some cases of acute colonic disease, however, a combination of histological features are pathognomonic of irradiation.

General Features of Radiation Injury

During the course of irradiation, a detailed light and electron microscopic study has shown no structural changes in the vasculature (Haboubi et al. 1988). This is hardly surprising because the endothelial cells are of intermediate sensitivity to radiation and, therefore, show no early changes. The presence of oedema in the lamina propria, which is a common phenomenon, may be related to either functional changes in the vascular endothelial cells, as has been suggested by Dewit and Oussoren (1987), or due to leakage from the damaged mucosal epithelium whereby luminal fluid transfers freely into the lamina propria. As we have not seen any damage to the vascular structure in early disease we would assume that leakage through the damaged epithelium is the more likely explanation. This concept is supported by the fact that oedema is not common in late disease despite the significant vascular damage. In late disease the epithelium is not significantly affected and therefore there is no increase in mucosal permeability.

After a few weeks or months, vascular changes appear and show features which explain many of the clinical aspects of the late disease. Similar structural changes

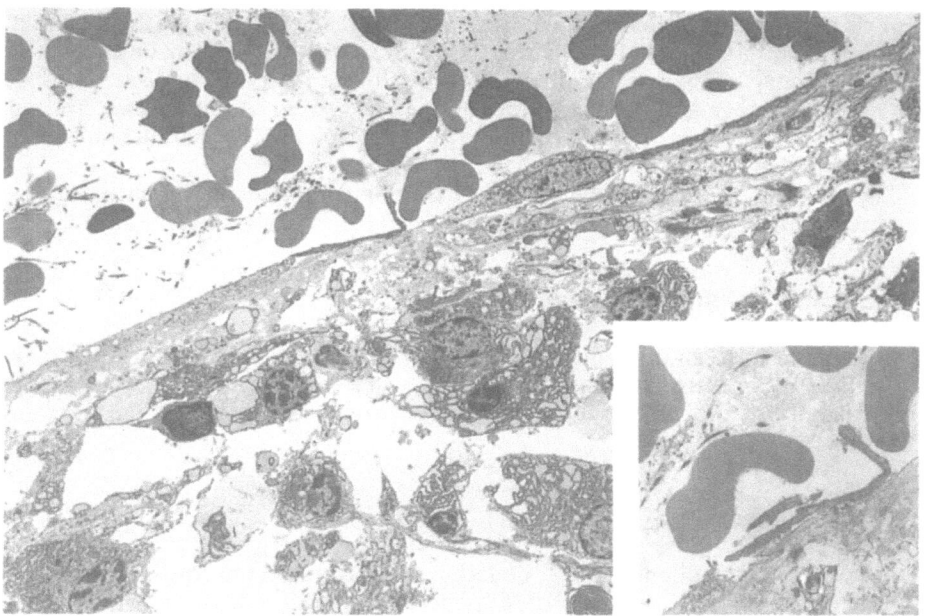

Fig. 2.2. Ultrastructural photographs of early degenerative changes within endothelial cell. Inset focal deposition of fibrin on "ulcerated" endothelial cytoplasm. Outside the vessels large numbers of inflammatory cells seen. (UALC × 1650, inset × 3250).

are seen in various target organs affected by late radiation disease. Thus, vessels of the urinary and gastrointestinal tracts show basically similar features. Vessels of all sizes, distributions and types are affected. These changes usually affect the entire vessel wall but always start with endothelial cell damage (Fajardo and Stewart 1973; Fonkalsrud et al. 1977). Ultrastructurally, these cells undergo a focal degenerative process leaving many cytoplasmic defects on which platelets and fibrin are deposited (Schofield 1987) (Fig. 2.2). Fibrin may occupy the lumen or extend outward to the damaged subendothelial layers to reproduce fibrinoid necrosis. The presence of thrombus reduces the blood flow but the thrombus also releases thromboxane, which leads to vascular constriction, further decreasing the blood supply to distal tissue.

In the capillaries the subendothelial damage is potentially more serious because of the lack of supporting tissue external to the endothelium. In the arterioles or arteries which have a scaffolding support of elastin, collagen, muscles and proteoglycans, the endothelial damage will deprive the inner third of the media of its nutrition (Crawford 1977). Whether this is the sole mechanism of medial damage or whether there is some direct effect of radiation is not certain. Both mechanisms may act independently or in combination.

In many cases, the vessels have transmural inflammation which may be florid. Fibrinoid necrosis and wall inflammation heal by fibrosis. Such scarred tissue cannot withstand the normal or increased local blood pressure which may lead to local aneurysm formation. In addition, it is possible that irradiation leads to fibrosis of the perivascular tissues which, with the passage of time, will retract. This retraction may actively "dilate" the vessel resulting in ectasia or aneurysm.

The vascular lumina which are blocked by thrombi may recanalise. Veins do not escape damage and show a variety of damage similar to the arteries. Intimal fibrosis, reduplication of elastic lamina and loss of media are all features of venous involvement.

The vascular damage produces three pathological processes which ultimately lead to a unified effect – tissue ischaemia.

Ectasia and Aneurysm Formation

This may not have an immediate effect but with the passage of time these weak-walled vessels yield to intraluminal pressure and expand and rupture. This leads to ischaemia of the tissues supplied by the vessels and to interstitial haemorrhages.

Occlusive Effect

This results from subendothelial oedema, fibrosis and from impacted thrombi (Hasleton et al. 1985). There is reduplication of the internal elastic lamina. Intimal fibrosis occurs in arteries and arterioles of all sizes. The percentage of mural arterioles with intimal fibrosis increases with time after radiotherapy. The thrombocytosis associated with radiation injury is a further factor encouraging thrombosis.

Arterial Medial Hypertrophy

The thickness of the media in non-irradiated tissue correlates with the diastolic blood pressure. There is increased medial thickness in arteries within irradiated bowel which is independent of blood pressure and age (Carr et al. 1988; Hasleton et al. 1985). It is believed that the increased thickness is due to the deposition of fibrin thrombi causing increased vascular resistance.

Ischaemia produces a characteristic tissue fibrosis. This is compounded by the healing of interstitial haemorrhages which result in further fibrosis. Vasculitis may produce a similar end-result. The fibrosis leads to further ischaemia due to obliterative vasculopathy, thus initiating a vicious circle. Ischaemia often produces segmental necrosis which plays a major role in fistula and abscess formation.

Pathology of Radiation Bowel Disease (Table 2.1)

Small Intestine

In conventional radiotherapy, the radiation is given in fractions and acute changes appear after each therapeutic dose and disappear soon after. The

Table 2.1.   Histopathology

Early radiation bowel disease	Late radiation bowel disease

Epithelial changes
  meganucleosis
  cell necrosis
  eosinophilic abscesses
	Epithelial changes
	  focal ulceration
	  branching crypts

Stromal changes
  eosinophilic infiltrate
  oedema
  fibroblastic reaction
	Stromal changes
	  vascular
	    ectasia
	    microaneurysm
	    thrombosis
	    xanthomatous reaction
	  fibrosis
	  haemosiderin

changes are always segmental and related to the continuous motility of the intestinal loops (apart from small segments of the terminal ileum, duodenum and upper jejunum). This motility protects any one area from receiving a critically high dose (Berthrong and Fajardo 1981). Therefore, in cases of pelvic irradiation the terminal ileum is more commonly affected whilst in upper abdominal irradiation the duodenum and upper jejunum show most of the pathology. If there are pre-existing peritoneal adhesions, motility is inhibited and no preferential protection of the intestinal loops can be expected (DeCosse et al. 1969). The small intestine is diffusely involved in cases of high dose whole body radiation. Sometimes an overwhelming and uncontrollable dehydration results due to loss of fluid and electrolytes secondary to extensive mucosal ulceration (Trier and Browning 1966).

Early Disease

The histological features of the early phase were described by Trier and Browning (1966). They found that within 12–24 hours of radiation, pyknosis and karyorrhexis appear in the crypts exhibiting cell death. As the crypt epithelium dies, there is a lack of cell replacement to the surface villi resulting in loss of mucosa and villous atrophy in 2–4 weeks. The lining surface cells become flat and focally ulcerated. These changes vary in intensity according to the location of the loop involved, the radiation dose and the time interval between the doses. After the full course and in mobile loops, the surface epithelium and the villi will be restored to normal in 2–3 weeks, while in fixed segments the recovery may be partial with persistence of villous atrophy and abnormally cystic crypts.

Late Disease

Gross Appearance. The gross appearance of the intestinal resectates in the late disease depends on the extent and duration of the disease. The serosal surface is thickened with fibrinous and/or fibrous plaques extending into the thickened mesentery. Commonly, several loops are matted together but rarely they are complicated by fistulae (O'Brien et al. 1987). The serosal changes have a haphazard arrangement with irregular patches and are never clean cut. Segments may show dilatation, variable lengths of stenosis or focal or confluent areas of transmural necrosis leading to irregular defects in the wall of variable sizes and shapes. In the stenotic segments the wall is markedly thickened by fibrosis mimicking the late stage of ischaemia or Crohn's disease. The muscularis stands out proud between the thickened serosa and submucosa. The mucosa almost always appears abnormal in areas of severe stenosis and may show typical cobblestone changes. Focal ulceration is common and can be seen at random or, more often, in relation to areas of severe fibrosis. These ulcers are invariably irregular, may be deep but more commonly are superficial.

Microscopic Features. The mucosa in irradiated areas almost always shows some abnormalities. The changes range from minimal flattening of the surface epithelium to shortening and thickening of the villi and marked reduction in inflammatory cells in the lamina propria. Submucosal oedema is prominent.

The crypts may be of normal size and shape or dilated and abnormal. The latter change is associated with fibrosis of the lamina propria. This fibrosis, characteristically glassy and homogenous, contains ectatic thin-walled vessels and atypical cells frequently termed "bizarre fibroblasts". These cells have not been identified immunohistochemically and could be derived from cells other than fibroblasts. Similar types of fibrosis are seen in the submucosa and serosa. Paneth cells are increased in number and the crypt epithelium shows an increased mitotic rate. The muscularis mucosa and propria are thickened in the stenotic segments of bowel. This is probably a compensatory hypertrophy for the loss of other muscle fibres. The vascular changes are seen throughout the wall and in particular in the thickened areas. In some cases the muscularis shows changes ranging from myocytolysis to frank infarction.

Large Intestine

Surgical pathologists see more specimens after resection for radiation injury of the sigmoid colon and rectum than the small intestine. Probably this is because the colon and rectum receive larger doses of radiation during treatment of pelvic malignancies and because the rectum is more fixed than the small intestine.

The basic pathological changes in the colonic wall are similar to the small intestine. The differences are mainly in the epithelial response because the colonic epithelium has a slower turnover rate (Williamson 1978) and more cells remain in the resting phase and are less susceptible to radiation.

Early disease is mainly an epithelial-type reaction characterised by meganucleosis, lack of mitoses, eosinophilic infiltration with the formation of eosinophilic abscesses and focal fibroblastic reaction in the lamina propria. These changes appear within days of radiation (Haboubi et al. 1988). Late disease occurs a few months later and is the fibrovascular phase of the disease. There is focal or diffuse vascular endothelial degeneration with formation of fibrin thrombi and accompanying fibrosis. The late effect of the disease can be divided into two main categories: the common ischaemic fibrosing stenosis and the rare neoplastic change.

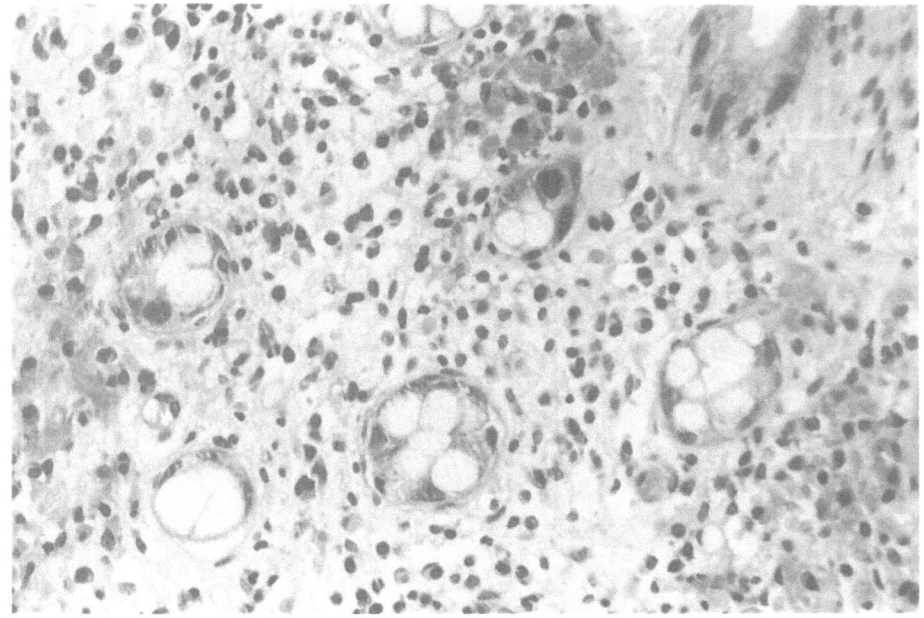

Fig. 2.3. Early large bowel disease. Some of the nuclei are massively enlarged in comparison with others in the same gland. There is no crypt distortion. (H&E ×150).

Early Disease

Although the colonic mucosal cells are "less active" than the small intestine enterocytes in turnover they are easier to study in the acute phase because of accessibility. The most significant histological features in the acute reaction are the following:

Nuclear Changes. (a) *Meganucleosis* is patchy and variable but seen in most cases. Cells both in the surface epithelium and the crypt are affected. The affected nuclei are large, 2–10 times the normal size (Fig. 2.3). They have either irregular "smudged" chromatin with irregular nuclear membranes or smooth enlarged open nuclei with prominent nucleoli. They occupy at least half the cytoplasm which is usually devoid of mucus. Meganucleosis represents a cell with a short-term high metabolic rate (Scarpelli and Chiga 1977). (b) *Lack of mitotic activity* is a uniform feature and is characteristic of the acute reaction. Radiation inhibits mitosis and DNA synthesis. The end result is a diminution of cell population (Rubin 1984).

Significant Eosinophilic Infiltrate. This affects the surface epithelium, the crypts and the lamina propria in up to 60% of cases with frequent pure eosinophilic abscesses (Fig. 2.4), (Haboubi et al. 1988). Some eosinophilic infiltrate is seen in most inflammatory processes of the colon but after radiation it assumes a large proportion of inflammatory cells. The actual cause of this reaction is not well known (Gelfand et al. 1968) but the presence of a similar infiltrate in the late

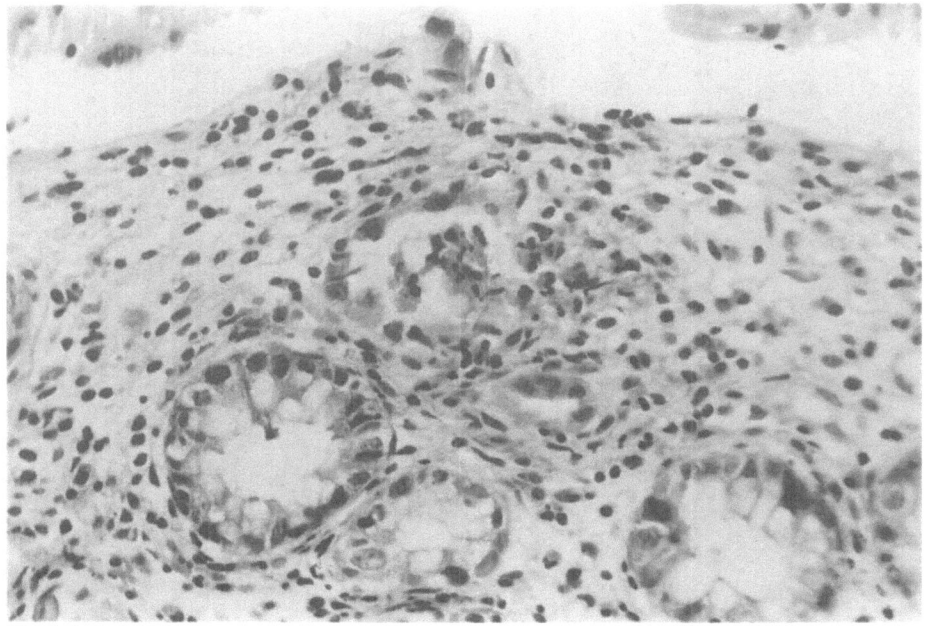

Fig. 2.4. Early large bowel disease. The lumen of one crypt contains groups of eosinophils forming eosinophilic micro-abscesses. Note that some glands show meganucleosis. (H&E ×250).

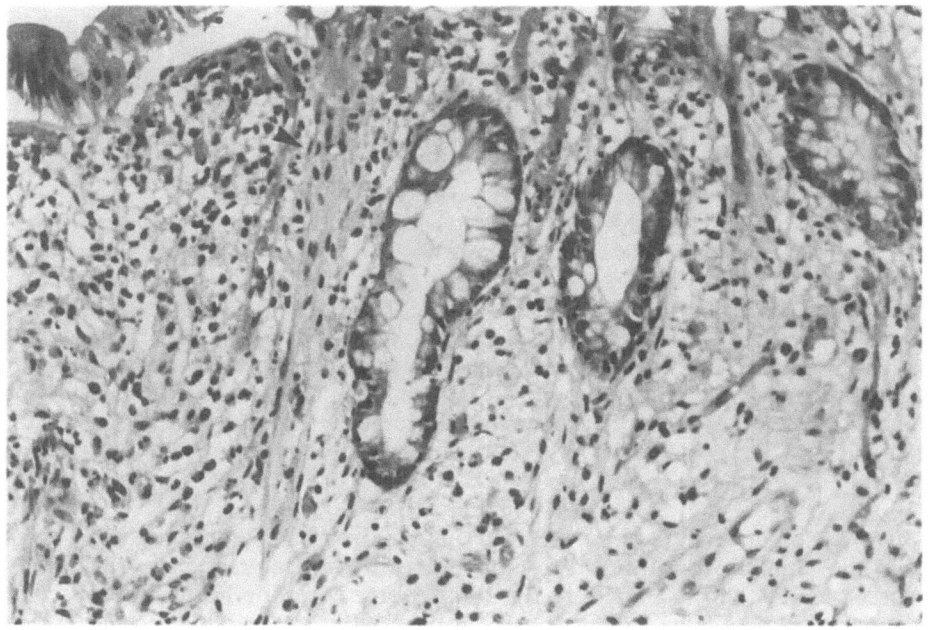

Fig. 2.5. Early large bowel disease showing oedema of the lamina propria and few fascicles of active fibroblastic proliferation (*arrowhead*). (H&E ×70).

disease suggests that the initial radiation insult has led to antigenic change of the epithelial cells to which eosinophils are reacting (Hasleton et al. 1985).

Fibroblastic Reaction. In about 30% of cases there is patchy but significant fibroblastic reaction seen in the lamina propria between and around the deeper crypts (Fig. 2.5).

Submucosal Oedema. Oedema of the lamina propria is commonly seen. On occasions this oedematous fluid extends into the crypts to produce subnuclear vacuolations.

Vascular Changes. At this stage no vascular changes are encountered.

The ultrastructural features support the light microscopic findings. The nuclei are enlarged, with smooth nuclear membranes. Some of the cells, either individually or in groups, show features of degeneration manifested by cytoplasmic condensation, lack of organelles or focal dissolution of the cytoplasmic membranes. In cases where there is extensive subnuclear vacuolation demonstrated on light microscopy, the ultrastructural changes show extensive displacement of the epithelial crypt cells by extra- and intracellular fluid (Fig. 2.6). The microvilli are not affected.

In the lamina propria there is an excess of proliferating active fibroblasts. These cells have prominent rough endoplasmic reticulum and mitochondria and are

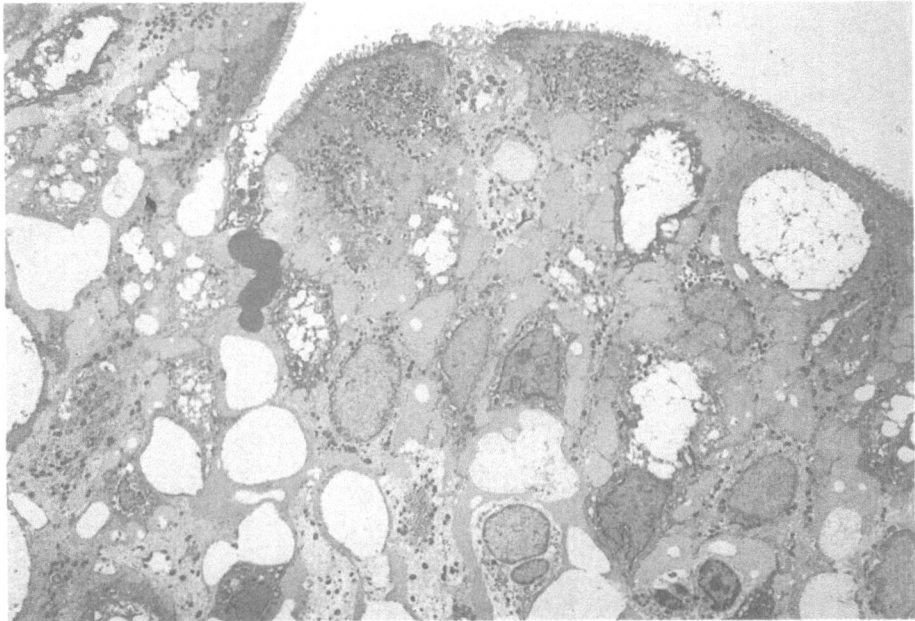

Fig. 2.6. Early large bowel disease showing the ultrastructural change in the crypts. There is marked displacement of the glandular cells by mostly extracytoplasmic fluid. The microvilli are intact. (UALC ×1180).

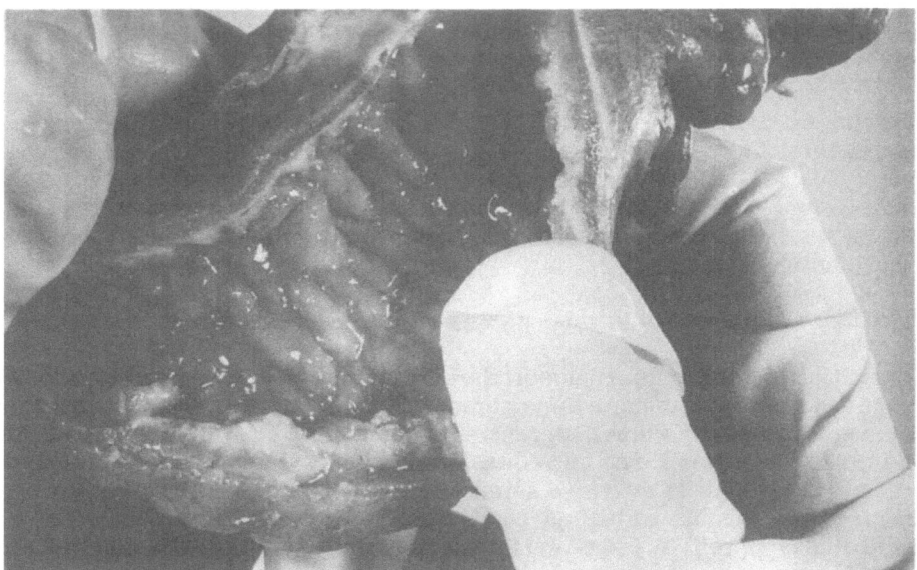

Fig. 2.7

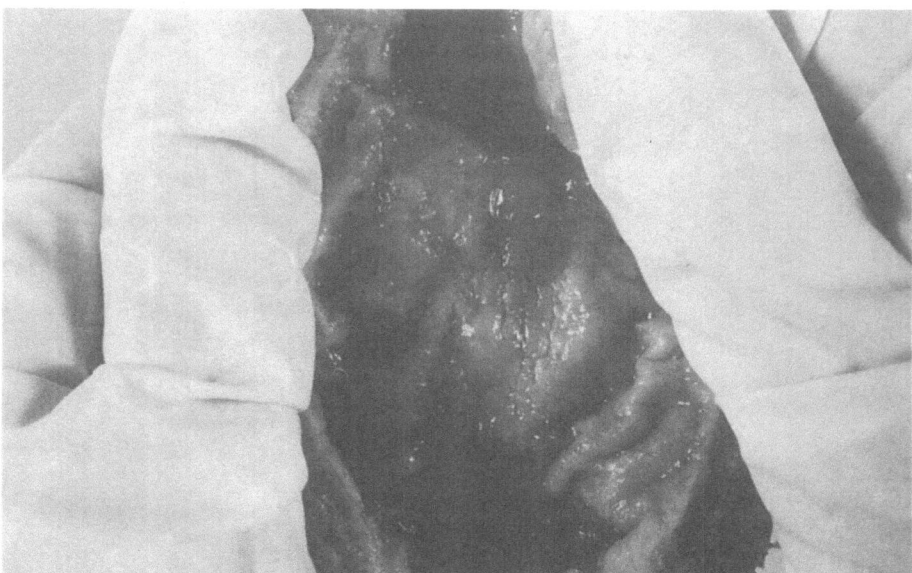

Figs. 2.7. and 2.8. Two cases of late radiation disease of large bowel showing the varied macroscopical appearances. In Fig. 2.7 there is cobblestone formation and the wall is focally thickened due to transmural fibrosis. Fig. 2.8 shows flat and featureless mucosa.1

surrounded by fine bundles of collagen. The blood vessels show no significant abnormality.

Late Disease

This is characterised by (a) predominance of the fibrovascular changes which are typical of this change and (b) the epithelium being relatively spared but with focal or confluent ulceration and crypt distortion. Neoplastic transformation is rare.

Gross Appearances. The macroscopic appearances reflect the ischaemic, fibrotic process. There is distortion of thickened, congested portions of bowel which are often matted together and characteristically have dull serosal surfaces. Fistula formation and ulceration are common features. The mucosa away from the ulcers is either oedematous and cobblestone in appearance (Fig. 2.7) or flat and featureless with frequent superficial or deep ulceration (Fig. 2.8). The wall is thickened and it may be difficult to distinguish its various layers.

Microscopic Features. The epithelial changes of meganucleosis and individual cell necrosis seen in the acute reaction are conspicuously lacking, reflecting the remarkable ability of these cells to regenerate. The persisting feature from the acute phase is the eosinophilic infiltrate though eosinophilic abscess formation is less frequent. The crypts are severely distorted, varying in size and shape and often appear branching. Paneth or pyloric cell metaplasia are not uncommon features.

   In the lamina propria there is a severe degree of hyalinised glassy fibrous tissue, a decrease in the normal lymphoid cell population and vascular damage. This type of fibrosis together with vascular changes and the presence of some bizarre or atypical mesenchymal cells distinguish the chronic reaction from Crohn's disease or pure ischaemia. The fibrosis which extends from the lamina propria to the muscularis propria and the serosa is of similar glassy appearance. The muscularis is often hypertrophied. The vascular changes are constant features and can be seen throughout the wall. The fibrous tissue is composed of mature, hyalinised thick bundles of collagen with few active fibroblasts. Nerves and ganglia are not affected.

Pathogenesis of Late Radiation Bowel Disease

It is difficult to predict which patients receiving radiation therapy will progress into chronicity. We believe that sequential biopsies may identify a common histological denominator in the early phase which will predict this progress. As a tentative hypothesis it is suggested that the subgroups of patients who develop early fibroblastic changes or eosinophilic abscesses may be most at risk. These may be indicators of potential progress to significant vascular damage. Once the train of vascular damage is set in motion it leads to ischaemia and fibrosis and may eventually produce necrosis with fistula and abscess formation. In some patients the ischaemic injuries may be minor but lead to very late presentation with a stricture or with malabsorption.

The second important but rare complication of late disease is the development of neoplasia. The tumour is invariably an adenocarcinoma with no distinguishing histological features from any ordinary adenocarcinoma. The latent period for the development of tumours may be up to 40 years after the initial exposure. A plausible explanation for this change is that clones of neoplastic cells may have arisen from an aberrant or mutant cell and many years later develop into the clinical carcinoma.

A curious and interesting but rare finding in the late disease is colitis cystica profunda. This was first noted by Black et al. (1980) in experimental animals but is also seen occasionally in humans (Gardiner et al. 1984). Large numbers of normal or dilated crypts are seen deeply seated at the muscularis propria. The normal and benign-looking cytological appearance and benign surface epithelium should differentiate this condition from carcinoma. The cause of this disorder is ill understood.

Urinary Tract Injury

Early urinary tract disease is very common but it is transient and rarely biopsied. As is the case with chronic radiation changes in general, late disease is mainly of fibrovascular origin and characterised by progressive fibrosis and a variety of vascular changes. Both elements may promote each other. In this phase the epithelial damage is minimal in most areas but localised necrosis may occur. There is frequent squamous metaplasia and occasional epithelial inclusions are seen deep in the muscular layer. The fibrous reaction has a characteristic histological appearance and distribution, particularly around nerve bundles.

Ureter

Early Disease

The availability of ureteric tissue from biopsies for early disease is very limited and autopsy studies suffer from the inevitable autolysis which affects mainly the mucosa. For these reasons the experience of ureteric injury in early disease is very scanty.

Late Disease

Gross Appearance. The lower part of the ureter is often thickened, firm and stenotic. The thickness and firmness are entirely due to extensive fibrosis. The surrounding soft tissue is also involved in the fibrotic process and adhesions are common. Proximal to the stenotic segment, ureteric dilatation is sometimes seen.

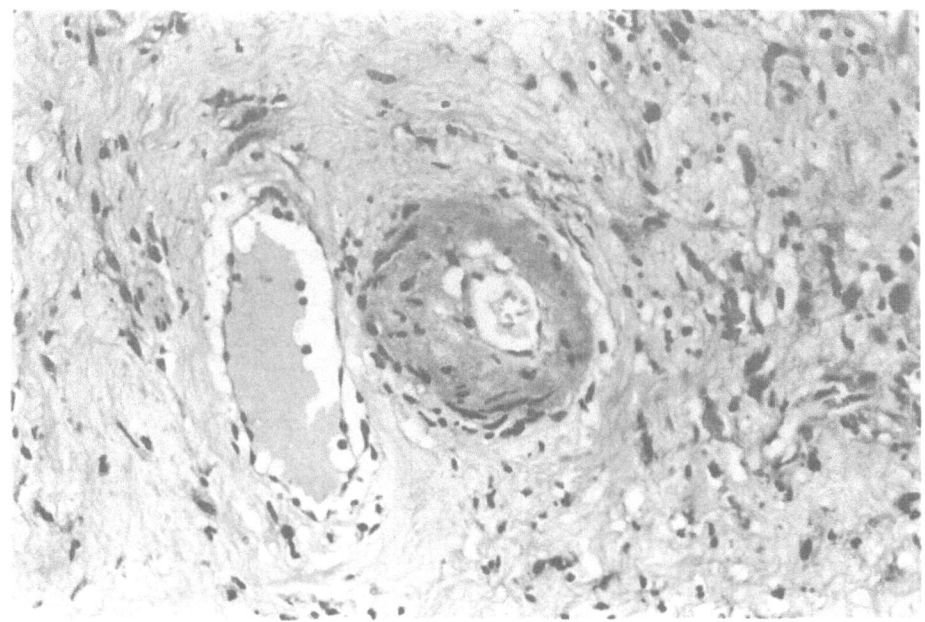

Fig. 2.9. Photomicrograph of a case of late ureteric disease showing a thickened artery and a dilated vein embedded in a fibrotic stroma. Subendothelial xanthoma cells are seen. (H&E ×110).

Total wall necrosis and fistulae such as uretero-vaginal or uretero-uterine are seen rarely.

Microscopic Features. With late disease, the most salient features are lack of epithelial damage and mild fibrosis which is mostly seen in the serosa, subintima and, rarely, transmurally. There is also vascular damage which is focal and minimal but can show the spectrum of changes which is seen in other organs (Fig. 2.9). Rarely, epithelial inclusions are found in the muscularis as well-formed dilated epithelial glands, characteristically surrounded by loose stroma with or without muscle fibres. Similar inclusions have been described in the large intestine of man and experimental animals, but not previously in the urinary tract. The possible explanations are:

1. Mucosal herniation due to increased intraluminal pressure. A similar feature is seen in diverticular disease of the colon.
2. Mucosal herniation due to active withdrawal of some parts of the mucosa by retractile fibrosis.
3. Misplacement of the glands during the regenerative process after ulceration. Some glands may be misguided or misplaced after the initial ulcerative process. This is akin to the situation in colitis cystica profunda and the term "ureteritis cystica profunda" is appropriate (Fig. 2.10).

Sometimes there may be subintimal, subserosal or transmural inflammation which, like the fibrosis, is minimal. Unlike the gastrointestinal tract, there is no

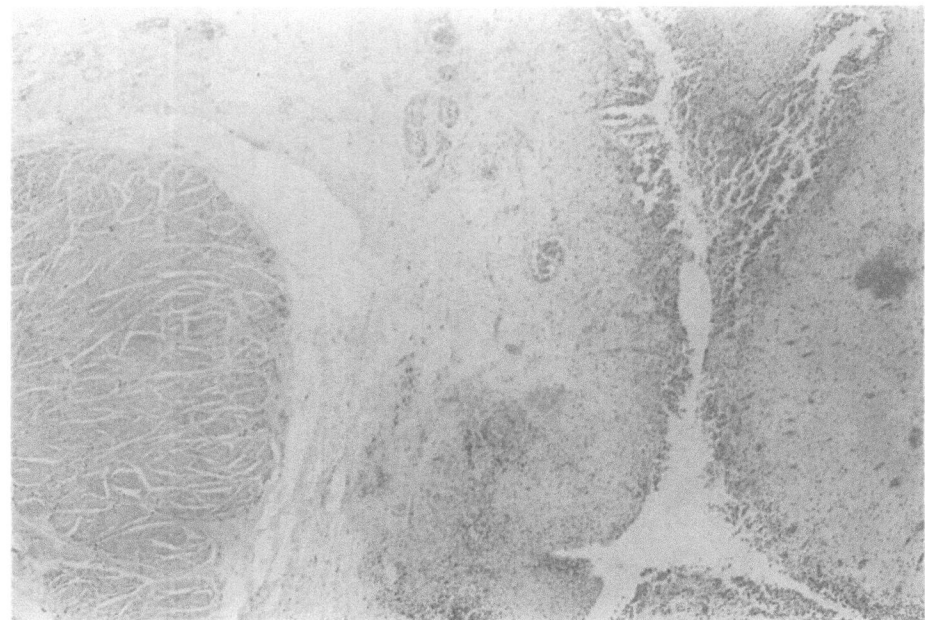

Fig. 2.10. Photomicrograph from a case of late radiation ureteritis showing deep invagination of the ureteric epithelium to form ureteritis cystica profunda. (H&E ×30).

specific predilection for eosinophils. The inflammatory cells are composed of plasma cells, lymphocytes and a few mast cells. In cases of ulceration neutrophils appear and predominate.

Bladder

Early Disease

As with the ureters early changes in the bladder due to irradiation are transient, thus rarely requiring active investigation. It is therefore unusual to have material for pathological assessment.

Late Disease

The morphological changes in the bladder are generally more severe than in the ureters. This could be due to an adverse interaction of the urine constituents and the damaged mucosa. Another factor may be the relatively high radiation dose to the bladder but the reason is uncertain.

Gross Appearances. Late disease may manifest itself months or years later and is characterised by haematuria, bladder contracture or necrosis (Wallace 1959).

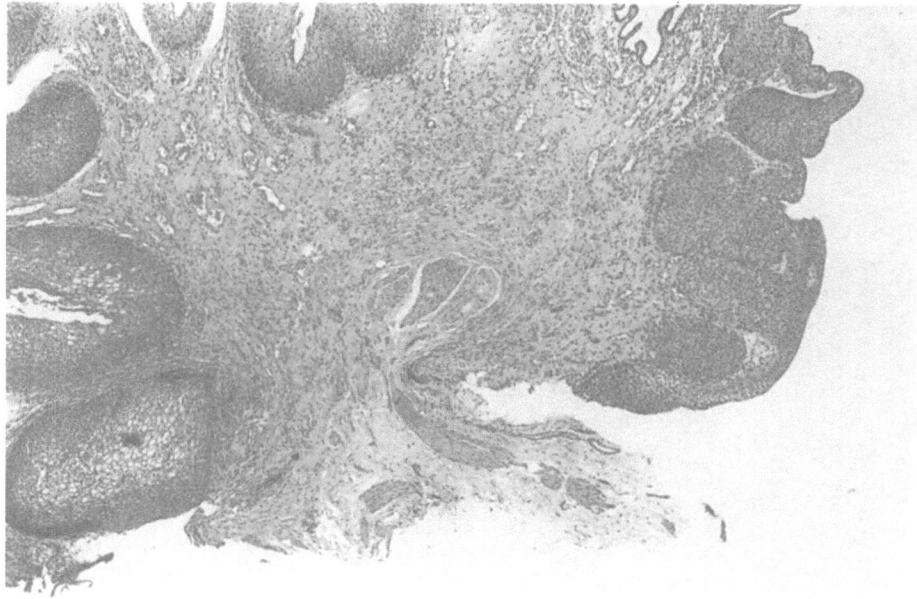

Fig. 2.11. Late radiation cystitis showing diffuse squamous metaplasia of the vaginal (glycogenated and clear cell) type. (H&E ×20).

The bladder is shrunken and fibrotic. The mucosa shows hyperaemic ulceration chiefly on the posterior wall above the interureteric bar. Occasionally ulceration is covered by a greyish membrane (Villasanta 1972). The contraction of the wall is due to extensive fibrosis of all the layers. In extreme cases the bladder has been described as a "thimble bladder". Full-thickness wall necrosis is a less common feature which may lead to vesico–vaginal fistulae or rarely to more complex fistulae.

Microscopic Features. The mucosal changes include diffuse or focal ulceration. The ulcers have no specific histological characteristics but occasionally include calcified particles. The intact epithelium does not show atypia or loss of polarity but there is occasionally mild meganucleosis. Sometimes diffuse squamous metaplasia of the vaginal type is seen (Fig. 2.11). This change may extend into the von Brunn's nests. This metaplastic process has been described by Neemann and Limas (1986) to affect only neoplastic bladder tissue after irradiation but in our experience, and in that of others (Pugh 1977), it is seen in previously non-neoplastic mucosa.

The fibrosis in the bladder has a characteristic appearance in type, distribution and cell constitution. As in the gastrointestinal tract the fibrous tissue is glassy, hyalinised and homogenous. It contains cells which are both mononuclear and multinucleated. The mononuclear cells may be large, polygonal or spindle, with open or hyperchromatic nuclei. The multinucleate cells are small or occasionally plump with closed lumina (Fig. 2.12). The number of nuclei varies from 2 to 6.

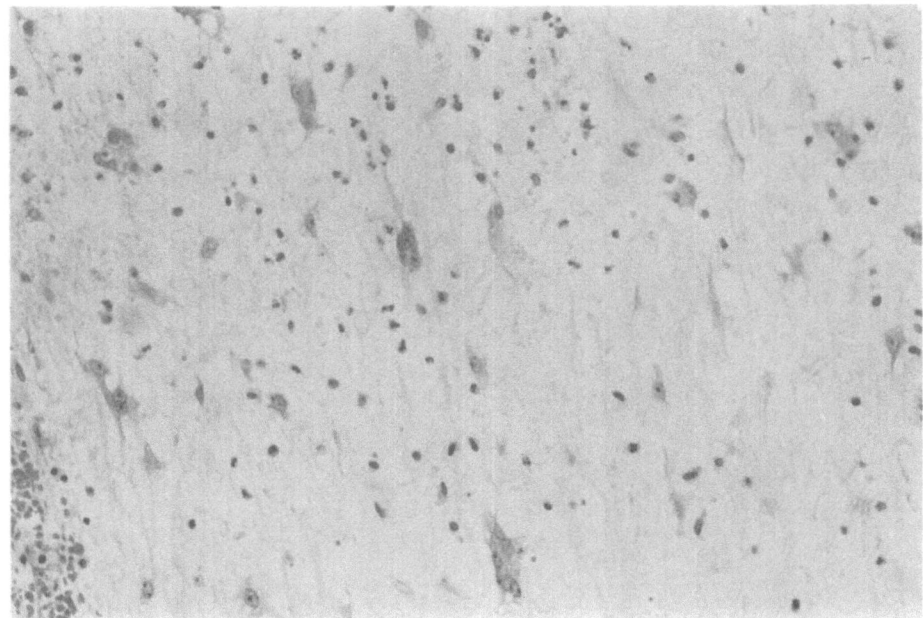

Fig. 2.12. Mono and multinucleated "stromal" giant cells in a case of late radiation cystitis.

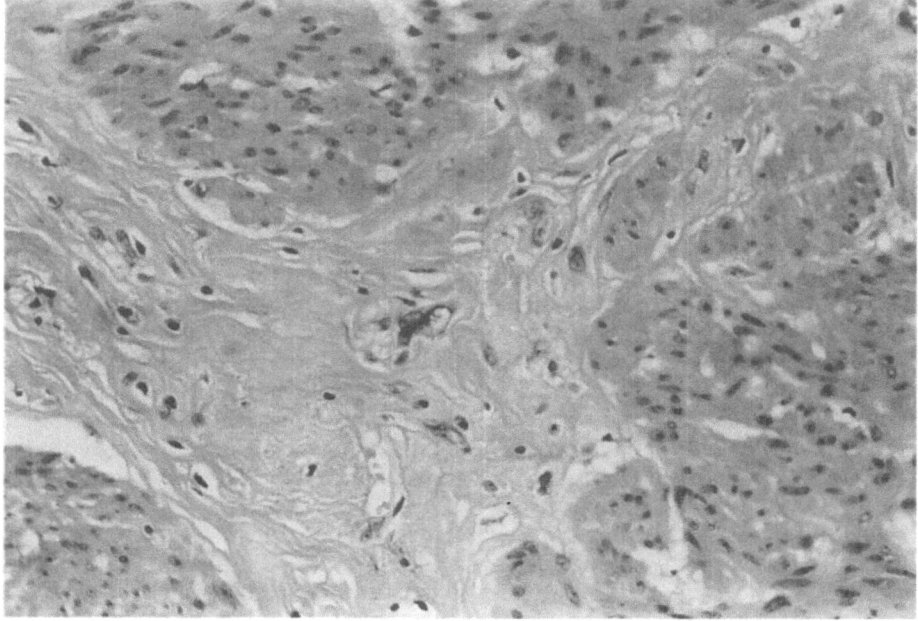

Fig. 2.13. Late radiation cystitis showing hyalinised dense fibrous tissue separating the bladder muscle. (H&E ×60).

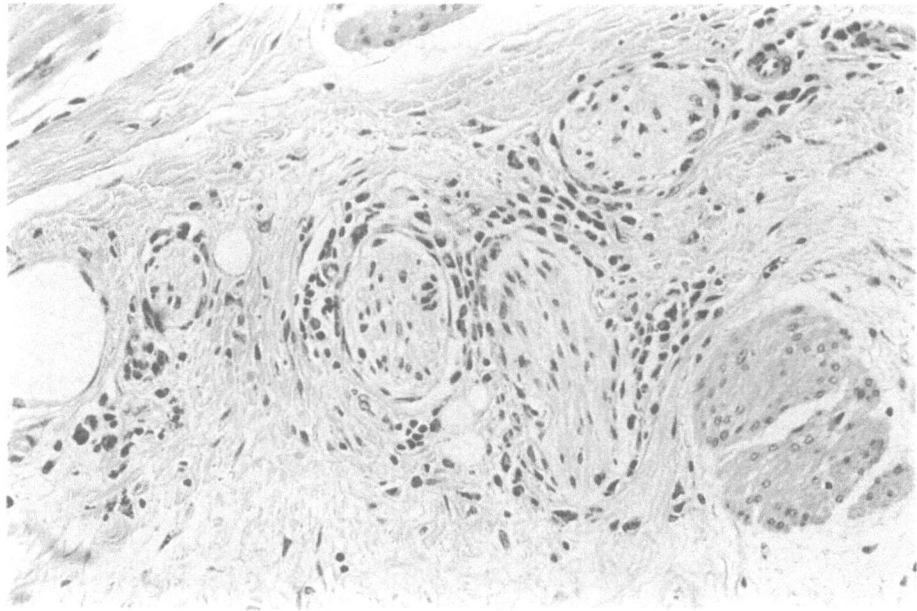

Fig. 2.14. Characteristic perineural fibrosis and mononuclear infiltrate in a case of late radiation cystitis. (H&E ×70).

The actual nature of the above types of cell commonly seen in the late disease has not been critically evaluated and further investigation is required to disclose their origin and significance.

The distribution of the fibrosis is of special interest. In addition to the subintimal and serosal fibrosis there are fibrous bands which separate the muscle fascicles into well-identified compartments (Fig. 2.13). There is often distinctive perineural fibrosis where nerve bundles are encroached upon or totally surrounded by well-organised fibrous tissue. This could be part of the generalised fibrous process or a localised nerve sheath reaction. The perineural fibrosis has a characteristic lymphoplasmacytic infiltrate (Fig. 2.14). If this type of fibrosis compromises the function and survival of the nerve bundles, it may directly compromise the contractility of the bladder. Occasionally, focal dystrophic calcification may be found, mostly in the areas of fibrosis or necrosis.

The vasculitis and vascular ectasia in the mucosa and submucosa may result in haematuria, to which these patients are particularly prone. If these changes occur elsewhere in the wall, intramural haemorrhages lead to haemosiderin deposition. There is often a marked but patchy deposition of haemosiderin seen through the bladder wall (Fig. 2.15). These haemosiderin deposits are sometimes accompanied by inflammation but are always seen in sites where the vascular changes are at their maximum.

Vascular changes in late disease have the same range of characteristic appearances as described earlier. The larger vessels, in particular the arterioles and arteries, suffer from vasculitis, luminal occlusion by fibrosis and sometimes

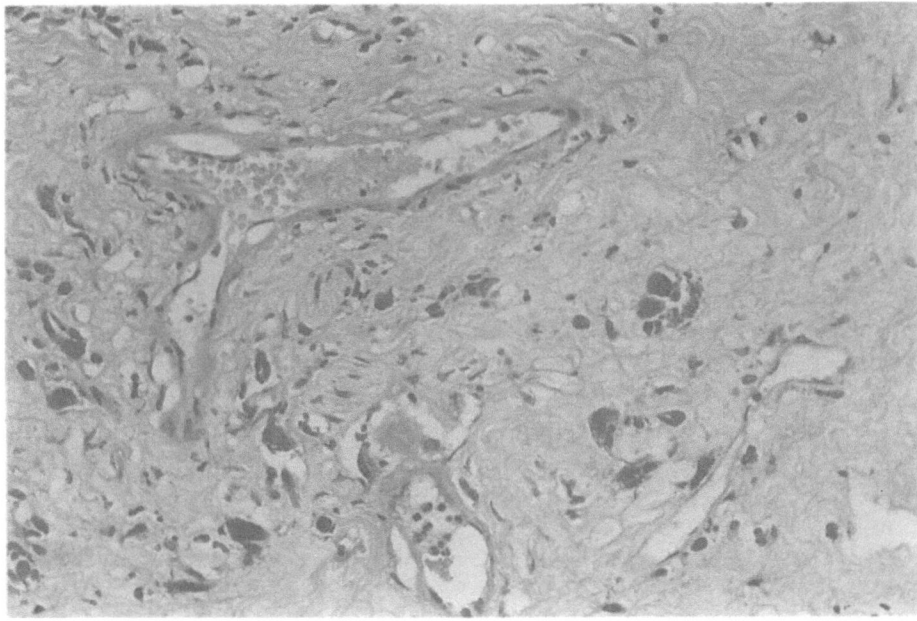

Fig. 2.15.   Ectatic thin-walled blood vessels embedded in dense fibrous tissue which contains large clumps of haemosiderin (late radiation cystitis). (H&E ×60).

subendothelial xanthomatous reaction. They are also occasionally mildly aneurysmal. The smaller vessels like the capillaries and the post-capillary venules become dilated.

The other important yet not pathognomonic feature is muscular hypertrophy. This is possibly related to the ischaemic effect produced by the fibrosis and luminal narrowing of the arteries. A similar phenomenon has been seen in ischaemic heart disease and it was thought to be due to compensatory hypertrophy for dying or non-functional muscular fascicles.

The histological changes seen in late disease of the urinary tract are summarised in Table 2.2. These changes taken together are characteristic and should not be confused with other conditions such as tuberculosis, schistosomiasis and other

Table 2.2.   Late urinary tract disease

Epithelial changes
   Squamous metaplasia
   Ureteritis and cystitis cystica profunda

Stromal changes
   Glassy, hyalinised fibrosis containing bizarre cells
   Perineural fibrosis
   Muscular hypertrophy
   Vascular changes
   Intramural haemosiderin deposition

---

specific inflammatory processes. There are some similarities between the late disease and burnt-out interstitial cystitis (personal experience). The similarities lie in the distribution of the fibrous tissue between the muscle fibres and the muscular hypertrophy. There are, however, more differences than similarities between these two conditions.

References

Berthrong M (1986) Pathological changes secondary to radiation. World J Surg 10:155–170
Berthrong M, Fajardo LF (1981) Radiation in surgical pathology, part 2, alimentary tract. Am J Surg Pathol 5:153–178
Black WC, Gomez LS, Yukas JM, Kligerman MM (1980) Quantitation of the late effects of X-irradiation on the large intestine. Cancer 45:444–451
Carr ND, Farragher EB, Hasleton PS (1988) Quantitative study of internal, longitudinal smooth muscle in human small mesenteric arteries. Acta Anat 32:69–73
Crawford T (1977) Blood and lymphatic vessels. In: Anderson WAA, Kissane JM (eds) Pathology, 7th edn. Mosby, St Louis, pp 879–921
DeCosse JJ, Rhodes RS, Wentz WB, Reagan JW, Dworken HJ, Holden WD (1969) The natural history and management of radiation-induced injury of the gastrointestinal tract. Ann Surg 170:369–384
Dewit L, Oussoren Y (1987) Vascular injury in the mouse rectum after irradiation and cisdiammine-dichloroplatinum. Br J Radiol 60:1037–1040
Fajardo LF (1982) The pathology of radiation injury. Masson Publishing USA, Inc, New York, p 6
Fajardo LF, Stewart JR (1973) Pathogenesis of radiation-induced myocardial fibrosis. Lab Invest 29:244–257
Fonkalsrud EW, Sanchez M, Zerbuarel R, Mahoney A (1977) Serial changes in arterial structure following radiation therapy. Surg Gynecol Obstet 145:395–400
Gardiner GW, McAulieffe N, Murray D (1984) Colitis cystica profunda occurring in a radiation-induced colonic stricture. Hum Pathol 15:295–298
Gelfand MD, Tepper M, Katz L, Binder H, Yesner R, Flouch M (1968) Acute radiation proctitis. Gastroenterology 54:401–411
Haboubi NY, Schofield PF, Rowland P (1988) The light and electron microscopic features of early and late phase radiation-induced proctitis. Am J Gastroenterol 3:1140–1144
Hasleton PS, Carr N, Schofield PF (1985) Vascular changes in radiation bowel disease. Histopathology 9:517–534
Neemann MP, Limas C (1986) Transitional cell carcinoma in the urinary bladder. Effect of pre-operative radiation on morphology. Cancer 58:2758–2763
O'Brien PH, Junrette JH, Garner AJ (1987) Radiation enteritis. Ann Surg 53:501–504
Pugh RCB (1977) Lower urinary tract. In: Anderson WAA, Kissane JM (eds) Pathology, 7th edn. Mosby, St Louis, pp 977–998
Rubin P (1984) Late effects of chemotherapy and radiation therapy, a new hypothesis. Int J Radiat Oncol Biol Phys 10:5–34
Scarpelli DG, Chiga M (1977) Characteristic cell injury and errors of metabolism. In: Anderson WAA, Kissane JM (eds) Pathology, 7th edn. Mosby, St Louis, pp 90–147
Schofield PF (1987) Radiation damage to the bowel. In: Taylor I (ed) Progress in surgery, vol. 2. Churchill Livingstone, Edinburgh London, pp 142–156
Trier JS, Browning TH (1966) Morphological response of the mucosa of human small intestine to X-ray exposure. J Clin Invest 45:194–204
Villasanta U (1972) Complications of radiotherapy for carcinoma of the uterine cervix. Am J Obstet Gynecol 114:717–726
Wallace DM (1959) Tumours of the bladder. Livingstone, Edinburgh London, p 280
Williamson RCN (1978) Intestinal adaptation: structural, functional and cytokinetic changes. N Engl J Med 298:1393–1402

3. Radiology of Radiation Injury

P. M. Taylor, R. J. Johnson and B. Eddleston

Clinical assessment of patients with radiation damage to the intestinal or genitourinary tract can be difficult. The symptoms may be similar to those of recurrent tumour. Radiology can be useful to document the presence and extent of any abnormality and to attempt to distinguish between radiation change and tumour. The findings help optimal management and indicate the need for other investigations including the use of interventional radiological techniques.

Radiological Assessment: Methods of Investigation

Individual patients may require assessment of the small bowel, large bowel and urinary tract. Others may require investigation of only two of these areas. Assessment will depend on the patient's clinical status, the treatment options available and the experience of the referring clinicians. Each area is considered separately below and the organ specific investigations discussed. The role of ultrasound (US) and computed tomography (CT) is discussed at the end of this section.

Small Bowel

The patient previously treated for carcinoma of the cervix with radiotherapy who presents with an acute distal small bowel obstruction and no clinical evidence of pelvic recurrence is more likely to have radiation disease than tumour as the cause of her symptoms (Walsh and Schofield 1984; Yuhasz et al. 1985). If the patient is being treated by a surgeon experienced in these problems then plain abdominal radiographs may be sufficient for management and the decision to perform a laparotomy.

In the subacute or chronic situation where the patient has non-specific symptoms and findings, barium studies are required. The small bowel enema is the investigation of choice and the methodology is well documented (Miller and Sellink 1979; Nolan 1983). This enables maximum distension of the bowel allowing early stenosing lesions to be identified. Particular attention should be paid to small bowel loops within the pelvis and the terminal ileum. One of the earliest changes of radiation damage is fixity of the loops within the pelvis and this can be easily overlooked. The loops should be palpated and compressed in order to separate them and allow peristalsis to be assessed fluoroscopically.

Large Bowel

The conventional double contrast barium enema is the investigation of choice to assess the large bowel. Because the appearances of a post irradiation stricture can be confused with colonic spasm, a muscle relaxant such as hyoscine butylbromide or glucagon should be used. Adequate views of the sigmoid colon are mandatory and double contrast radiographs in differing degrees of obliquity should be obtained. A lateral rectal radiograph must be obtained to assess the pre-sacral space. The examination may need to be modified in individual patients to demonstrate complications such as recto-vaginal fistula, when erect views will be required. An external fistula is better demonstrated by a fistulogram using water-soluble contrast medium. Because of the risks of associated bacteraemia it is desirable that this procedure is covered by antibiotic therapy.

Urinary Tract

The intravenous urogram (IVU) is the most widely used investigation of the urinary tract. In our experience a drip infusion technique using 200–250 ml of contrast such as Urografin 150 (diatrizoate) or Omnipaque 140 (iohexol) given intravenously over a period of 10–15 minutes is the most satisfactory way to demonstrate the ureters. At the end of infusion a full abdomino-pelvic radiograph is obtained with further radiographs 10 and 20 minutes later. Localised views of the bladder when full and after micturition should be taken (Schenker 1964). In addition to these routine radiographs selected views or fluoroscopy may be necessary, for example to demonstrate a vesico-vaginal fistula or to project the lower ureter away from bone.

Although the density of the nephrogram is somewhat reduced by using this infusion technique it is not a problem in this group of patients. Abdominal compression is not used because one of the main indications for the examination is to identify ureteric obstruction. Our use of non-ionic or low osmolar contrast medium is confined to those patients considered at risk of an adverse reaction (Grainger 1984).

Dependent upon the findings on the IVU, other investigations may be required. If there is a non-functioning kidney an ultrasound examination will establish the presence of a kidney, its size and the degree of any dilatation of the pelvicalyceal system. If dilatation is present and the site of obstruction cannot be determined on the ultrasound scan an antegrade pyelogram, under ultrasound guidance, may be performed. This technique is well documented (Weinstein and Skolnick 1978) and will accurately determine the level of obstruction. If this is at a level above the radiotherapy field a post radiation stricture is excluded. The obstruction may be due to metastatic lymphadenopathy. If ultrasound has not demonstrated this, then a CT scan may support the diagnosis. Biopsy of the glands under CT or ultrasound guidance can be undertaken.

Demonstration of obstruction to the distal ureter within the radiotherapy field requires distinction between radiation damage and recurrent tumour. Decompression of the obstructed system by percutaneous nephrostomy may be necessary for pain relief, drainage of a pyonephrosis or recovery of function. If the obstruction is bilateral and associated with renal failure, global kidney function will be improved in most cases by undertaking a nephrostomy on one side only. Very occasionally bilateral nephrostomies are required when a unilateral nephrostomy fails to improve renal function. The degree of hydronephrosis, and where possible the results of an isotope renogram, help to establish the kidney most suitable for nephrostomy. Ideally the better-functioning kidney should be punctured. Care must be taken to avoid converting a chronically obstructed kidney into a pyonephrosis. Insertion of a ureteric stent through the obstruction, either antegradely by the percutaneous route or retrogradely at cystoscopy, may be required as a palliative procedure in those patients who are deemed unsuitable for surgery. Retrograde examinations are rarely undertaken to identify the site of obstruction because we feel that the combination of ultrasound and antegrade pyelography is preferable as the risk of infection is lower.

Divided renal function can be assessed by isotope renography. Our practice is to perform serial gamma camera renograms as described by O'Reilly et al. (1986), to provide objective evidence of deterioration in individual renal function due to progressive damage. The isotope renogram can also be useful in assessing the results of surgical treatment when the morphology demonstrated on the IVU may remain abnormal. Diuresis renography may be a useful adjunct to the conventional renogram in differentiating the dilated non-obstructed system from the actively obstructed kidney.

Ultrasound and Computed Tomography

Some of the indications for the use of ultrasound and CT have been referred to already. These techniques have a useful if limited role in the differentiation between radiation disease and tumour recurrence. Ultrasound can be used to assess the pelvic soft tissues. Bladder filling and emptying can be evaluated and this may be useful in the patient with a rigid fibrotic bladder wall complaining of frequency or incontinence. In addition the bladder wall thickness can be documented. Like the IVU its use in the demonstration of mucosal abnormalities is limited. It can be of value in the assessment of the cervix and parametrial tissues and may demonstrate tumour eroding through the posterior wall of the bladder (Fig. 3.1). Ultrasound can also demonstrate the presence of pelvic or para-aortic and para-caval lymphadenopathy. However, as it cannot characterise tissue, histology may be required from the enlarged nodes or abnormal parametrial masses because pelvic nodes may be enlarged due to the presence of infection or reactive hyperplasia rather than the presence of metastases. Likewise the parametrial tissues may be increased in size due to fibrosis, infection, tumour, or any combination of these. Metastases in normal-sized lymph nodes cannot be identified. Assessment of the retroperitoneum may be difficult or inadequate in obese patients or when the presence of bowel gas obscures this region. In the

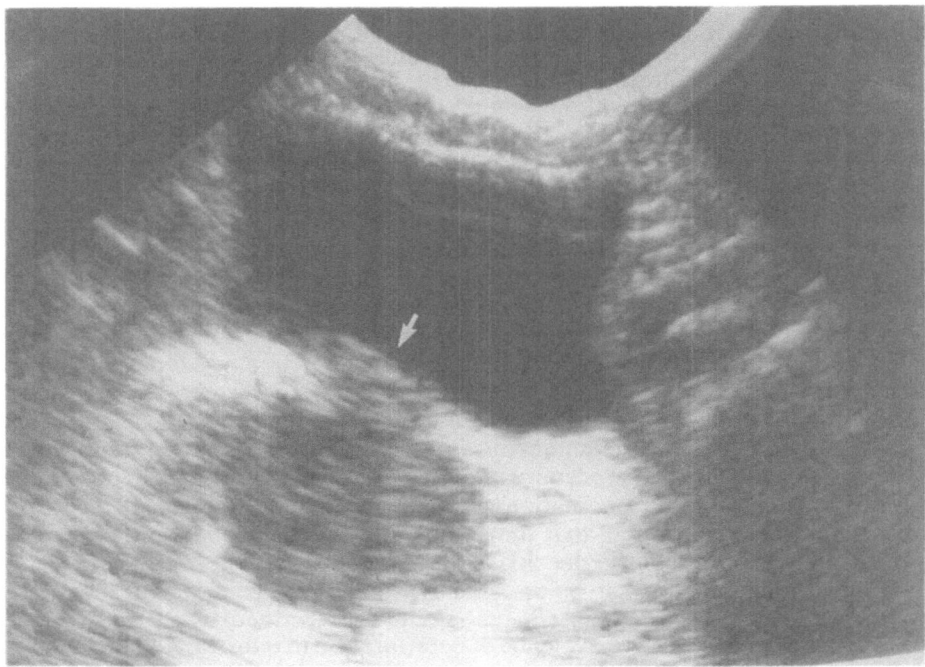

Fig. 3.1.   Transverse axial ultrasound scan demonstrating extension of carcinoma cervix through the posterior bladder wall (*arrow*).

presence of renal failure ultrasound is a valuable investigation, mainly to establish the likelihood of a post renal, obstructive cause for the failure. In practice, upper urinary tract obstruction producing renal failure is more commonly due to tumour recurrence than radiation disease.

CT is a non-invasive technique capable of providing an excellent demonstration of morphological changes within the pelvis and abdomen. There are limitations of its use related to its cost and availability and like ultrasound its inability to characterise tissue. This last limitation leads to similar problems to ultrasound in assessing parametrial masses and pelvic and abdominal lymph nodes. Retroperitoneal anatomy is better demonstrated than with ultrasound and the obese patient or the presence of bowel gas cause no problems. In the pelvis certain features characteristic of radiation damage can be identified. These include bands of soft tissue in the posterior pelvis (Fig. 3.2), thickening of the peri-rectal fascia and thickening of the bladder wall, occasionally associated with ulceration. Some of these features are not appreciated on ultrasound. An uncommon complication of radiotherapy is stenosis of the cervical os, with uterine enlargement due to a pyometrium. This can be diagnosed on ultrasound or CT (Fig. 3.3). Recurrent tumour, rather than radiotherapy change, as the cause of occlusion of the cervical os cannot usually be excluded by these imaging techniques. In our practice CT is found to be most useful in identifying and demonstrating bulk tumour recurrence with radiation damage being assessed by organ specific techniques.

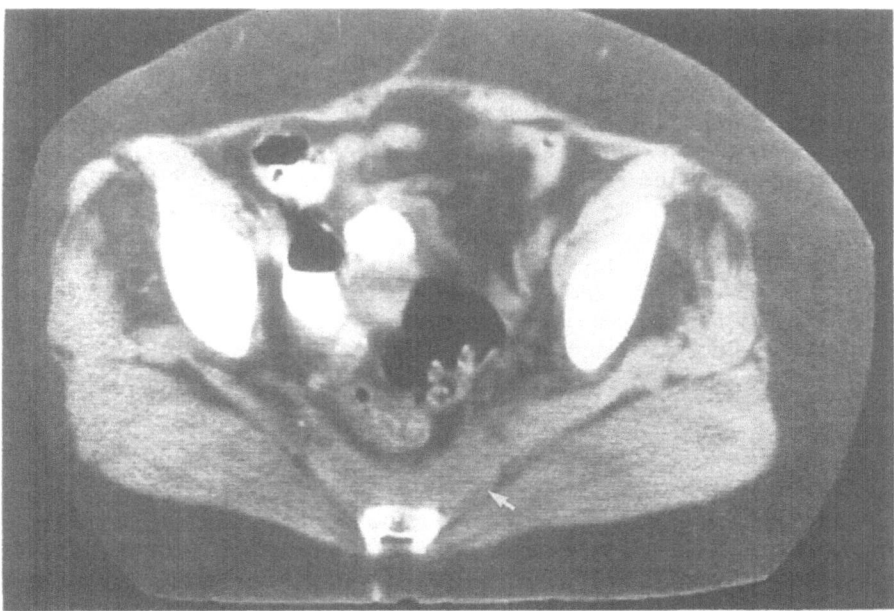

Fig. 3.2. CT scan demonstrating a band of soft tissue density in the posterior pelvis (*arrow*) due to radiation fibrosis.

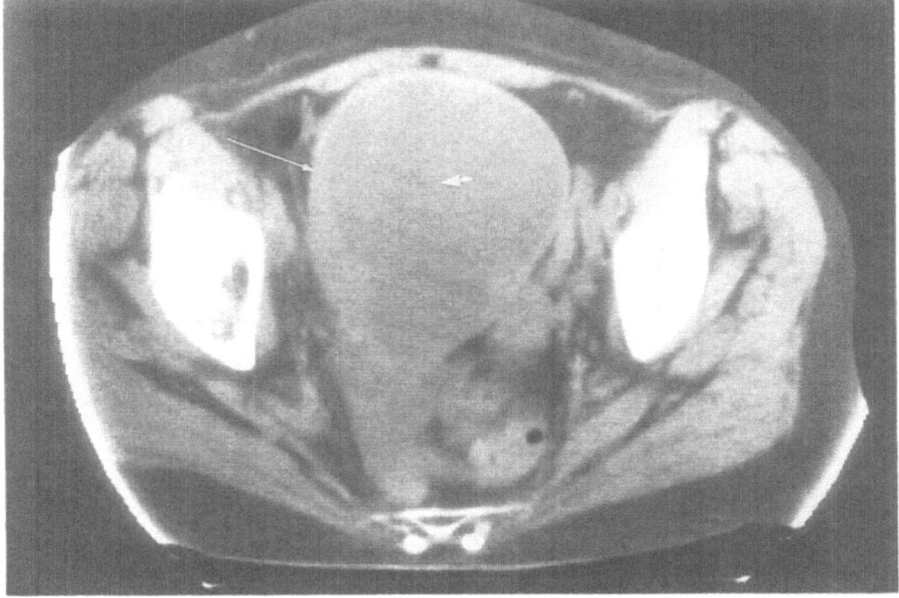

Fig. 3.3. CT scan demonstrating a large fluid collection within the endometrial cavity (*thick arrow*) which is distending the myometrium (*thin arrow*). At surgery this was a pyometrium.

Radiological Signs

One of the major problems encountered in the radiological assessment of radiation disease is the poor correlation which may exist between clinical signs and symptoms and the radiological findings. In the bowel the lack of gross mucosal changes may make a radiation lesion difficult to recognise or may lead to an underestimate of the disease severity. Early ureteric strictures demonstrated on the IVU may produce few, if any, symptoms and no signs. Alternatively the patient may have chronic radiation cystitis producing haematuria and dysuria with extensive telangiectasia visible on cystoscopy but a normal IVU. This section describes the radiological signs in specific regions of interest.

Small Bowel

The two commonest investigations are the plain abdominal radiograph and the small bowel enema. The plain abdominal radiograph, which usually includes an erect or lateral decubitus view in addition to the supine view, can demonstrate features of distal small bowel obstruction (Fig. 3.4a,b). The features are non-specific except that the obstruction is usually incomplete with evidence of gas within the large bowel and no gross dilatation of the small bowel. This appearance

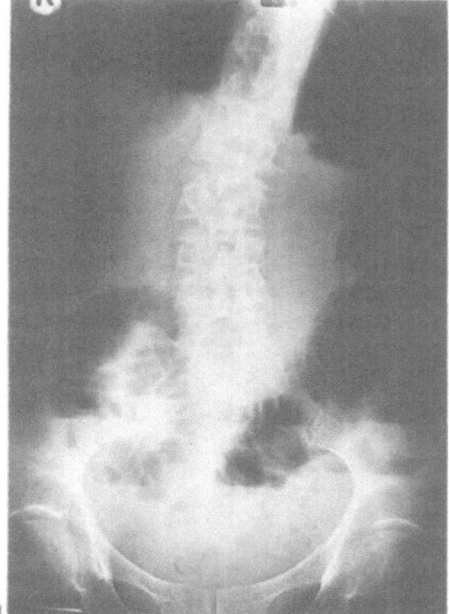
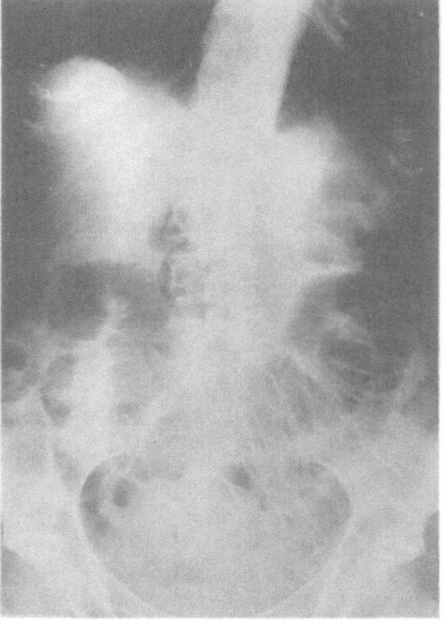

Fig. 3.4.a Erect and **b** supine abdominal radiographs demonstrating small bowel dilatation and multiple gas/fluid levels due to obstruction within the pelvis.

in a patient with carcinoma of the cervix treated with radiotherapy is presumed to be due to radiation damage unless there is clinical or radiological evidence of recurrent tumour. Radiological evidence of tumour recurrence includes demonstration of a central pelvic mass or lymphadenopathy on ultrasound or CT and bone erosion from adjacent lymphadenopathy. In contradistinction, small bowel obstruction in patients with ovarian carcinoma is usually due to recurrent tumour (Walsh and Schofield 1984; Yuhasz et al. 1985).

The radiological features of radiation damage seen on barium studies have been described previously (Mason et al. 1970; Rogers and Goldstein 1977; Mendelson and Nolan 1985) and are illustrated below from patients in our own series (see Appendix). Barium studies are often indicated in patients with chronic symptoms in whom surgery is contemplated as an elective procedure. In our experience they are only rarely required in the acute situation. Changes only occur in the small bowel that has been within the radiotherapy field and the commonest site is in the ileum. The changes are the result of fibrosis and necrosis due to radiation endarteritis (Hasleton et al. 1985), and may occur throughout the bowel wall. The mucosal folds become thickened and straightened and so the valvulae conniventes become more prominent (Fig. 3.5). Mucosal ulceration,

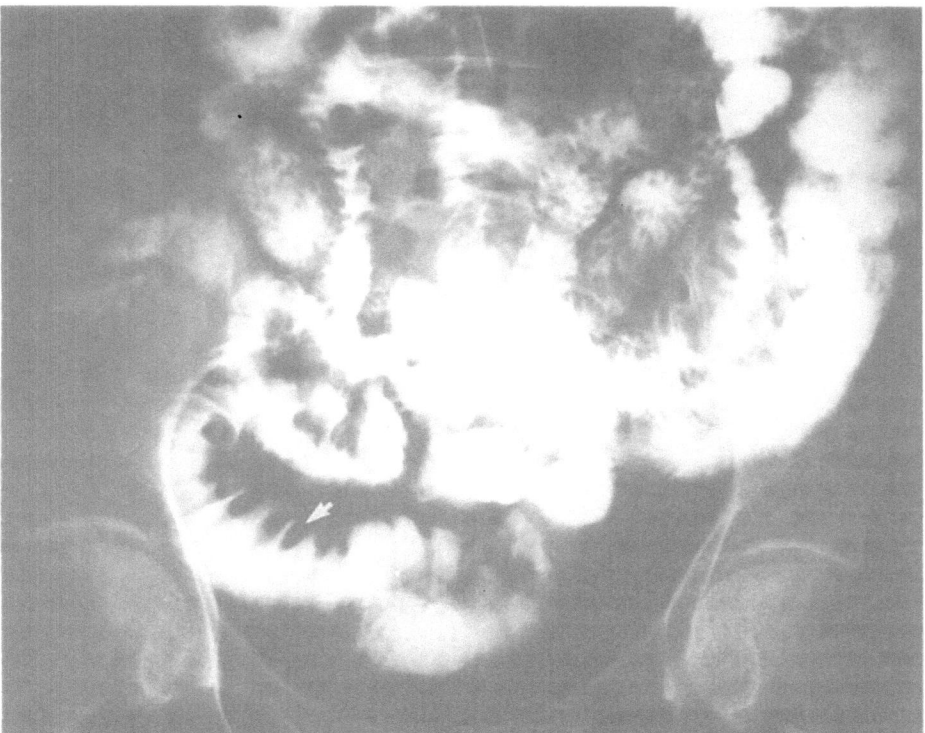

Fig. 3.5. Small bowel study demonstrating thickening and straightening of the valvulae conniventes (*arrow*) in a loop of ileum lying within the pelvis. Adjacent bowel loops are separated due to thickening of their walls.

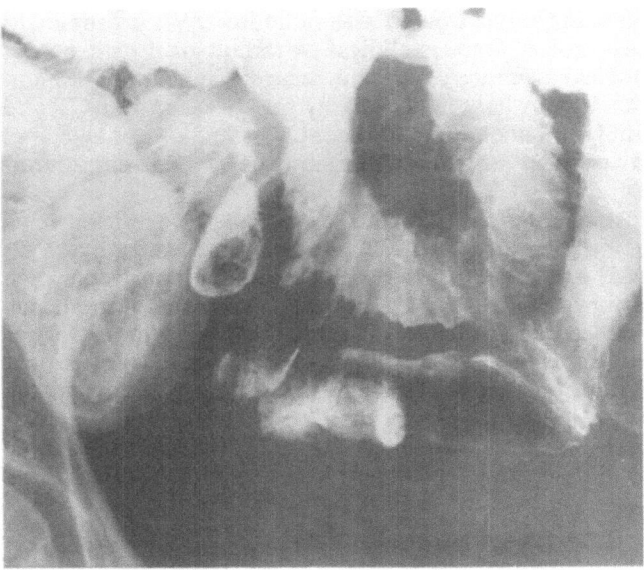

Fig. 3.6. Small bowel study demonstrating fixed and angulated ileal loops within the pelvis. Thickened valvulae conniventes are also seen.

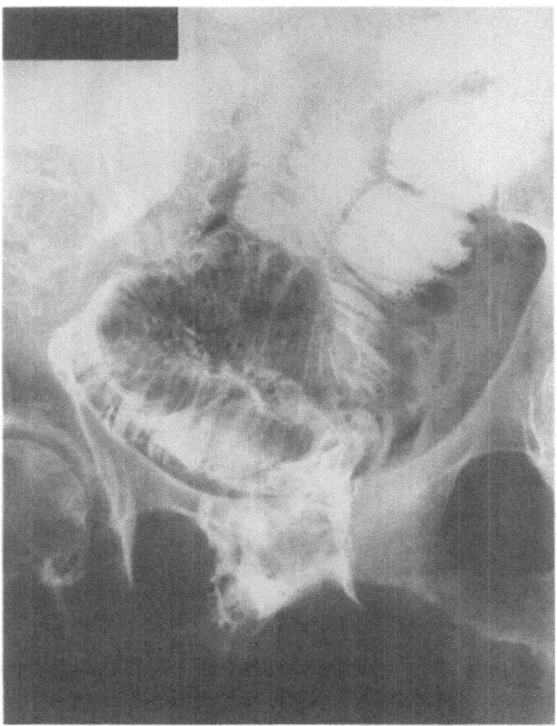

Fig. 3.7. Small bowel study demonstrating a fistula from the jejunum to the perineum.

which may be evident microscopically, is rarely seen radiologically (Mason et al. 1970; Rogers and Goldstein 1977). We failed to demonstrate ulceration in any patient. Some authors have described mucosal nodular filling defects or "thumb printing" (Mason et al. 1970; Rogers and Goldstein 1977). This is presumed to be the result of oedema and is similar to the appearances which may be seen in ischaemic bowel disease. No examples of this feature were seen in our own series. The fibrotic process leads to the bowel becoming thickened, rigid and immobile, with reduced peristalsis. Bowel loops may become fixed within the pelvis and demonstrate abnormal angulation (Fig. 3.6). It must be emphasised that the loops are palpated, compressed and examined fluoroscopically in order to identify early changes. The loops may become narrowed and stenotic but this is a late manifestation (Mason et al. 1970). Associated mesenteric fibrosis may cause traction upon the bowel loops and produce appearances similar to those seen in carcinoid tumours (Mendelson and Nolan 1985). The bowel loops may be separated from one another by thickening of the wall by fibrosis, or they may be matted together in an inseparable "mass" within the pelvis, the latter appearances being described as pooling (Mason et al. 1970). Spontaneous fistulae may occur between the skin or the large bowel or the genitourinary tract and the small bowel. A rare fistula to the perineum is shown in Fig. 3.7. There can be a narrowed segment of small bowel with smooth, featureless mucosa (Fig. 3.8). This is an unusual finding and dilated loops of small bowel are occasionally seen proximal to the damaged segment.

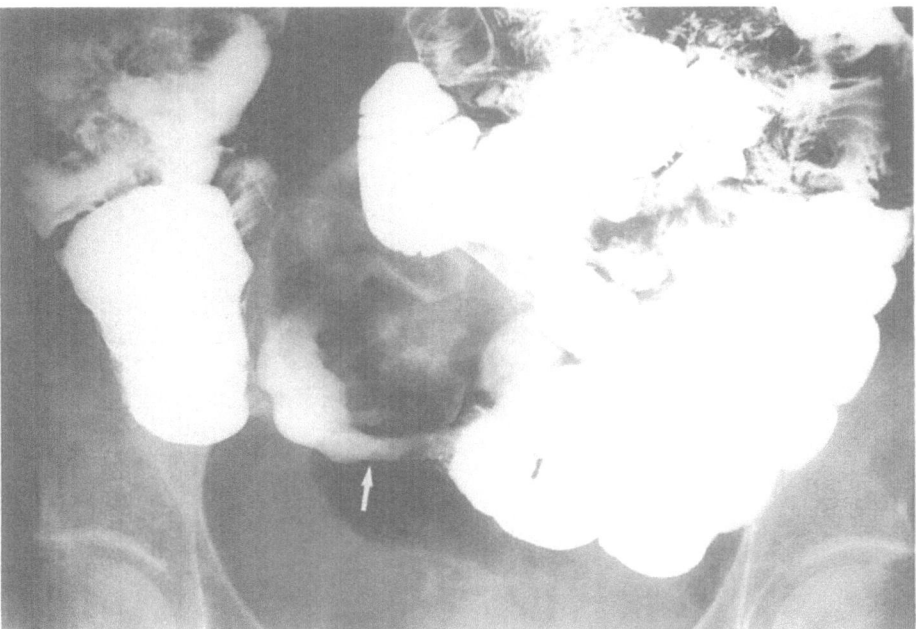

Fig. 3.8. Small bowel study demonstrating a narrowed loop with smooth, featureless mucosa (*arrow*).

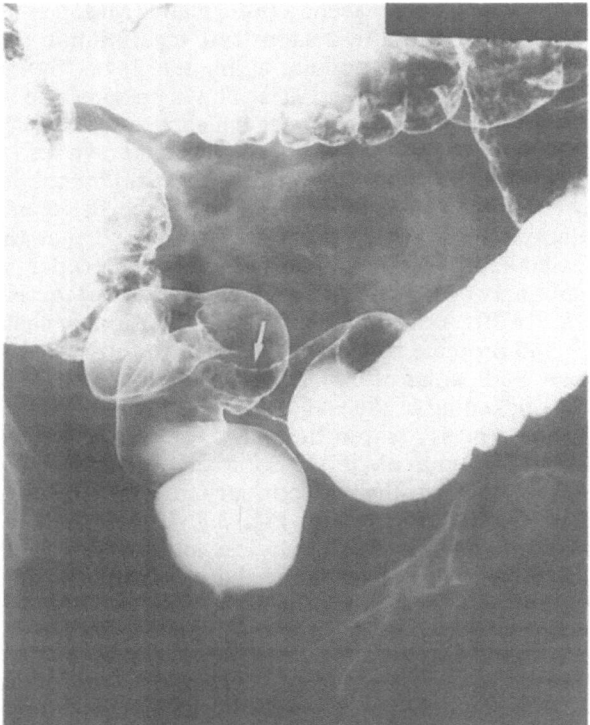

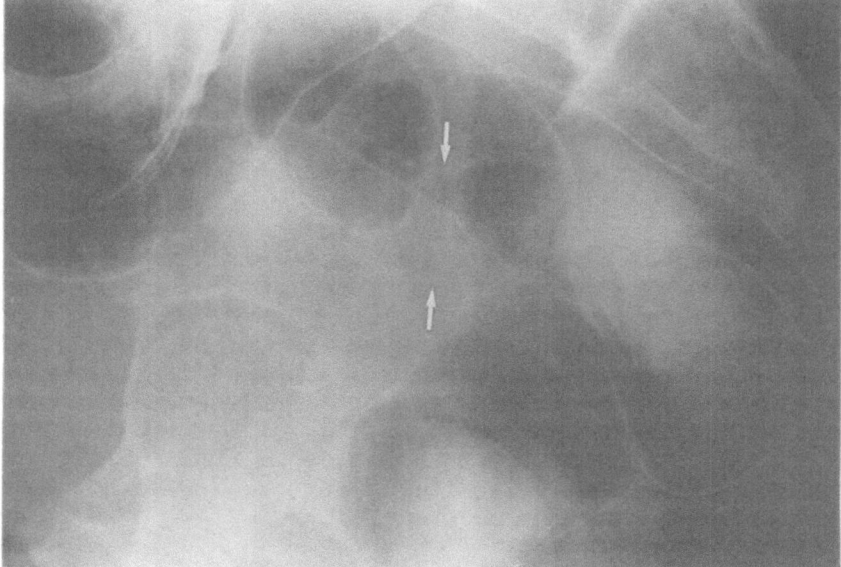

Fig. 3.9.a Double contrast barium enema (DCBE) demonstrating a smoothly tapered segment within the sigmoid colon (*arrow*). **b** DCBE with a less obvious area of radiation damage within the sigmoid colon (*arrow*).

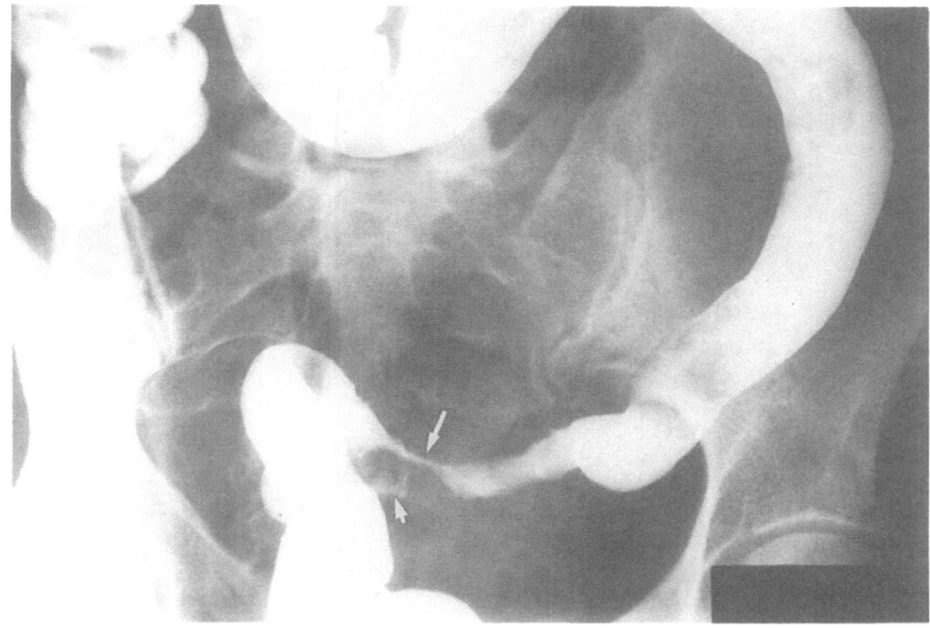

Fig. 3.10. Barium enema demonstrating a "stricture in a stenosis" (*long arrow*). This patient also demonstrates a fistula (*short arrow*).

Large Bowel

The commonest abnormality is a stricture which is typically a smoothly tapered lesion lying in the mid sigmoid colon or upper rectum. However its length, position and mucosal pattern can vary (Fig. 3.9 a,b). In our series the length varied from 3–30 cm. Some of these lesions were of an apparent "stricture in a stenosis" configuration in which a portion of colon was narrowed over a distance of several centimetres but within this was a much shorter segment of more severe stenosis (Fig. 3.10). Sometimes more than one area of narrowing is seen. Occasionally the stricture involves a continuous segment of upper rectum and sigmoid colon (Fig. 3.11 a,b). We observed one patient where a stricture in the sigmoid colon produced complete obstruction. She presented as an acute problem, the plain abdominal radiographs showing changes of distal large bowel obstruction, and a post irradiation stricture was found at emergency laparotomy.

Within the affected segment the mucosal pattern is characteristically effaced, becoming smooth and featureless. However, mucosal irregularity can occur and, in this regard, we have noted three principal patterns:

1. *Fine surface ulceration.* The appearances are similar to those seen in mild colitis with fine spiculations and loss of clarity of the mucosal margin (Fig. 3.12).
2. *Deeper focal ulcerations.* Although these are more commonly seen on sigmoidoscopy they are rarely demonstrated on barium enema (Fig. 3.13).

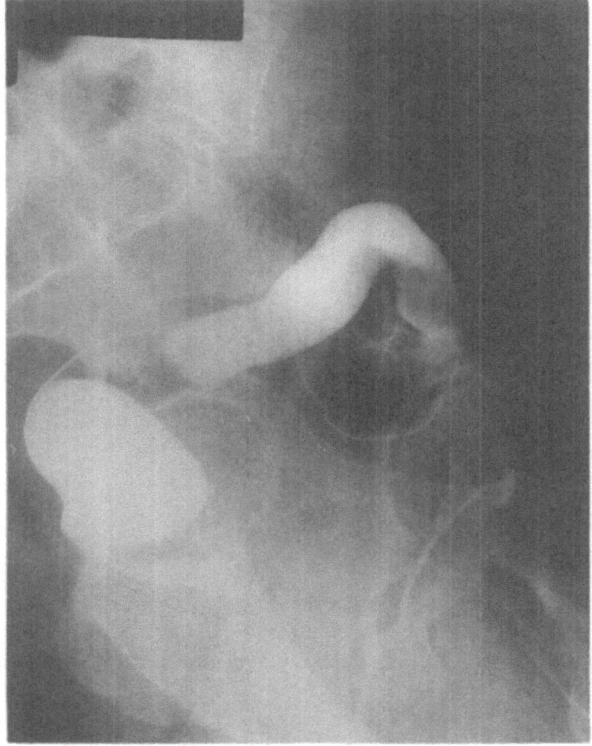

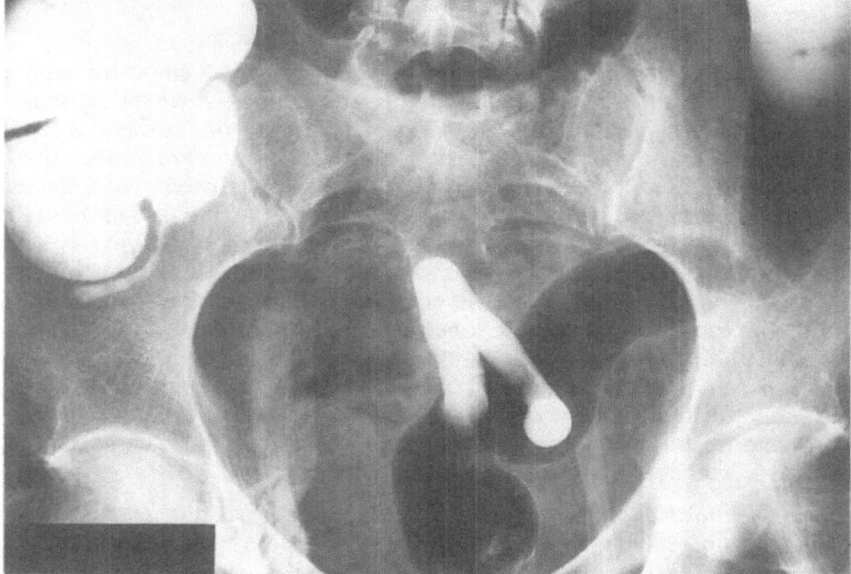

Fig. 3.11. DCBE in two patients (**a,b**) each demonstrating a continuous stricture of the upper rectum and sigmoid colon. **a** also demonstrates widening of the pre-sacral space.

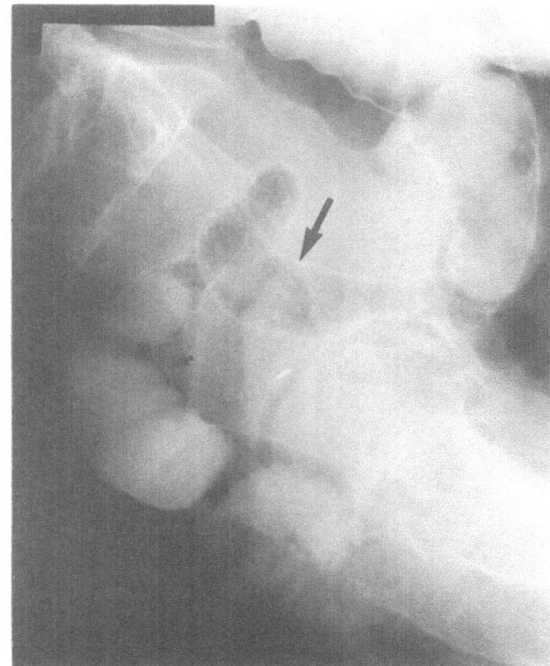

Fig. 3.12. DCBE. Fine surface ulceration. There is loss of clarity of the mucosa (*long arrow*) within the sigmoid colon when compared with the appearances in the rectum (*short arrow*).

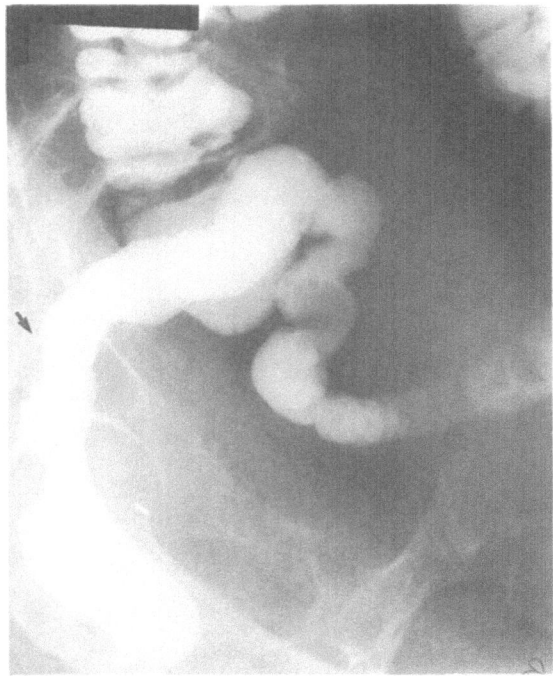

Fig. 3.13. Barium enema demonstrating focal ulceration in the upper rectum (*arrow*).

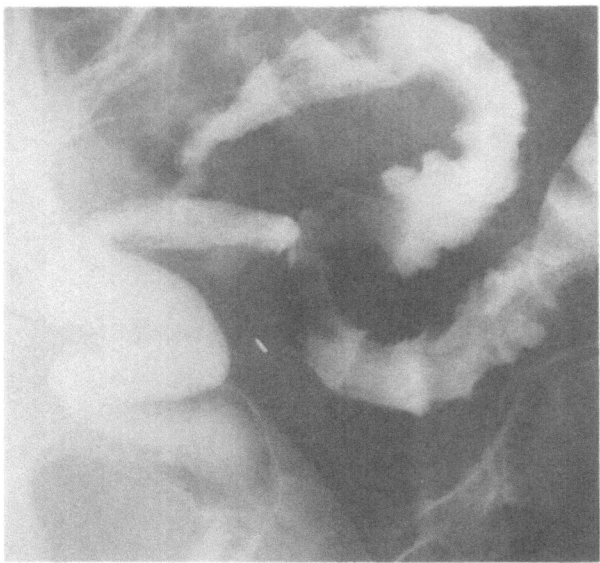

Fig. 3.14.

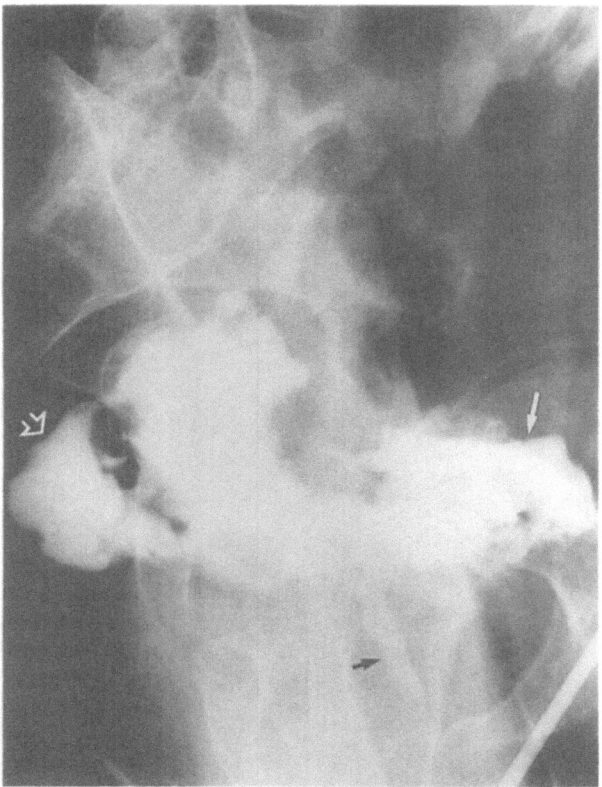

Fig. 3.15.

Fig. 3.14. DCBE demonstrating generalised mucosal thickening.

Fig. 3.15. Fistulogram. The patient is holding a Foley catheter in an osteum on the skin. Contrast is seen filling a large cavity which consists of the bladder (*thin white arrow*), vagina (*thin black arrow*) and rectum (*thick arrow*).

◄───

3. *Generalised mucosal thickening and irregularity.* This produces a "cobblestone" pattern with interlacing linear streaks of barium seen in fissures between the mucosal thickening (Fig. 3.14). These appearances can be similar to those described in Crohn's disease.

It is important to realise that the only abnormality may be a narrowed segment which retains a normal mucosal and haustral pattern. Like the small bowel the large bowel may become fixed and angulated but fixity is more difficult to appreciate in the large bowel. It may only be evident with repeat examinations when no appreciable change in the position of the lower sigmoid colon is seen.

A fistula may occur from the rectosigmoid region and most commonly involves the vagina or bladder. Occasionally a large fistula occurs leading to the formation of a single cavity comprising the rectum, vagina and bladder (Fig. 3.15).

Spasm has been documented as the earliest radiological abnormality (Mason et al. 1970). However spasm is a common feature of the normal barium enema examination and its presence is of little value in differentiating normal from abnormal. We would always recommend the use of a smooth muscle relaxant prior to the examination being undertaken. Extrinsic changes may affect the large bowel. The commonest of these is the development of peri-rectal fibrosis which causes traction on the rectum, resulting in its anterior displacement and widening of the pre-sacral space. This can be demonstrated on a lateral radiograph with barium in the rectum (Fig. 3.11a).

Two other features have been observed in individual patients, which were thought to be the result of radiotherapy. One patient appeared to have hypertrophy of the circular muscle in the proximal sigmoid colon in the absence of stricture or diverticular disease. We assume the distal sigmoid colon was more rigid than normal and the consequent rise in colonic pressure resulted in proximal muscle hypertrophy. In another patient with diverticular disease, several of the diverticula were flattened in appearance with angulated contours. In this case we assume the diverticula were bound down by peri-rectal fibrosis (Fig. 3.16).

Urinary Tract

As illustrated in the Appendix our own experience of urinary tract disorders after radiotherapy for carcinoma cervix differs from some descriptions – ureteric damage has been more common than in some other series (Slater and Fletcher 1971; Muram et al. 1981). The most frequent ureteric abnormality is a smoothly tapered stricture involving the lower ureter and extending proximally from the vesico-ureteric junction over a few centimetres (Fig. 3.17). The average stricture in our series has been 3 cm in length but we have seen lesions as long as 8 cm.

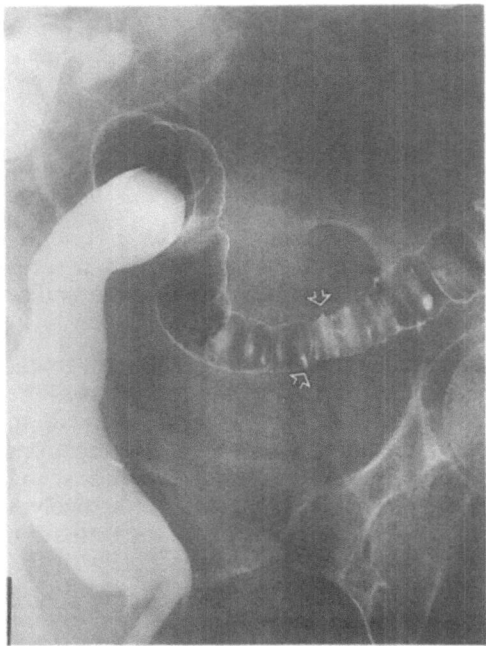

Fig. 3.16.   DCBE demonstrating diverticula modified by radiation damage (*arrows*).

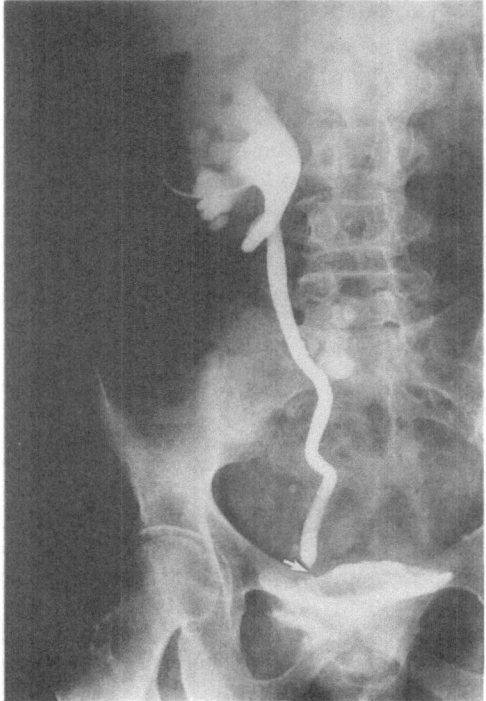

Fig. 3.17.   Antegrade pyelogram demonstrating a smoothly tapered distal ureteric stricture (*arrow*). The patient also has a vesico-vaginal fistula.

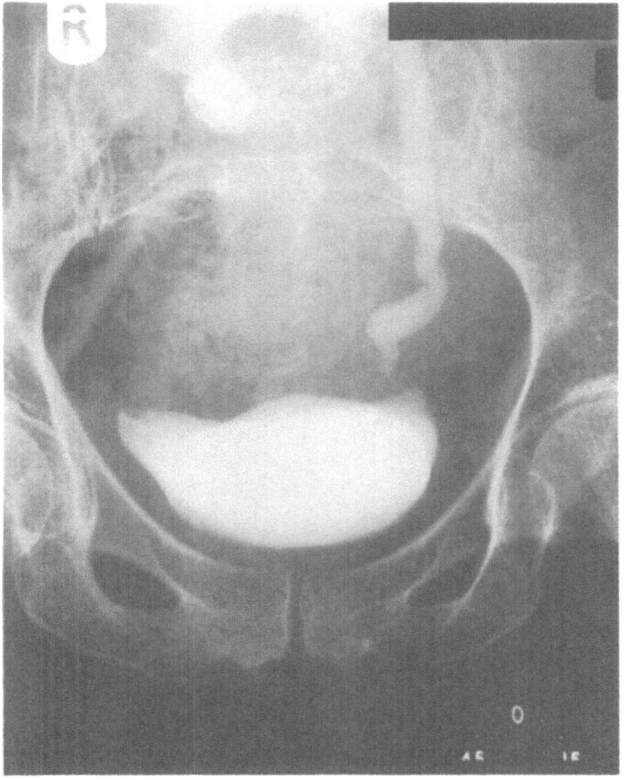

Fig. 3.18. Intravenous urogram (IVU) demonstrating a distal left ureteric stricture, found at post mortem to be due to tumour recurrence. The appearances are similar to those seen in Fig. 3.17.

The diagnostic problem is to distinguish post irradiation stricture from recurrent pelvic tumour. Our experience is that this is difficult and may be impossible. We have compared the appearance of radiation strictures with those due to recurrent tumour and were unable to demonstrate any differentiating features (Fig. 3.18). However the distinction between these two conditions is important and therefore histology is desirable. Ureteric strictures can be seen at the level of the pelvic brim with a normal distal ureter (Fig. 3.19). Previous authors have attributed this to the presence of metastases in the iliac nodes and adjacent ureteric involvement or compression by the large nodes. We have experience of four patients who all had surgical and histological evidence that such strictures were due to radiation damage. Therefore it is important that patients with high ureteric strictures have histological confirmation before they are diagnosed as having metastatic disease.

Fistulae from the urinary tract are less common than those from the intestine (Kjorstad et al. 1983). In our series one patient had a uretero-colic fistula, another a uretero-vaginal fistula. The uretero-colic fistula developed following a small bowel resection with freeing of the ureter from a fibrotic mass. The uretero-vaginal fistula was spontaneous.

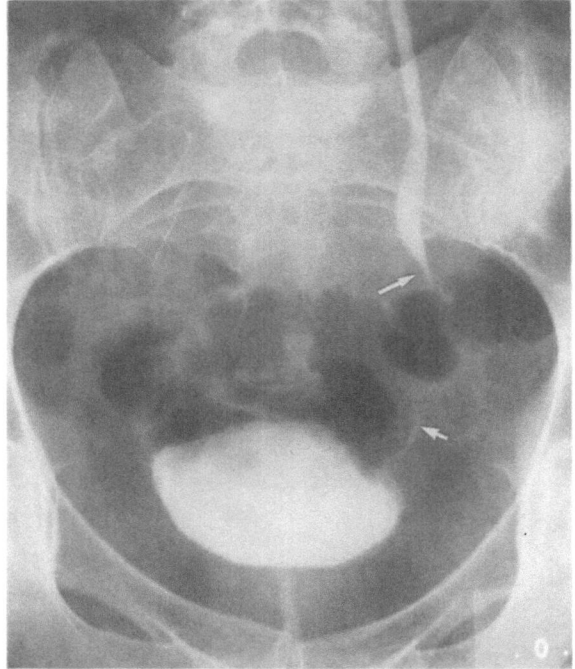

Fig. 3.19

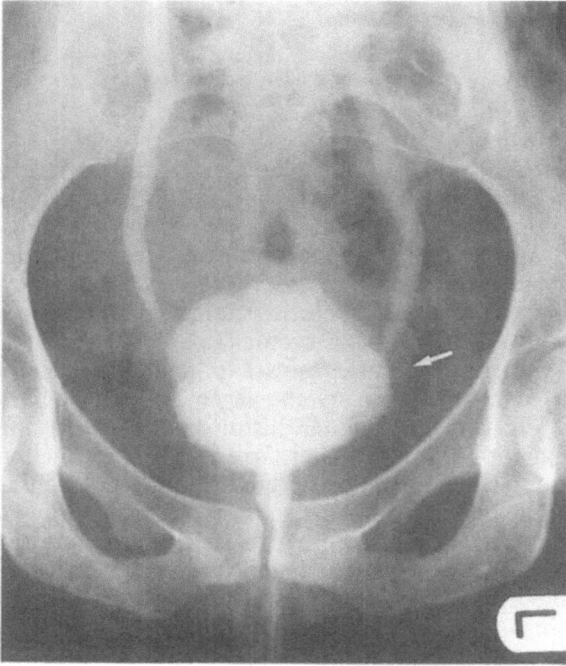

Fig. 3.20

Fig. 3.19. IVU demonstrating a left ureteric stricture at the pelvic brim (*long arrow*). A normal distal ureter is seen (*short arrow*). Histology confirmed the stricture was due to radiation damage.

Fig. 3.20. IVU demonstrating a small volume bladder with mucosal irregularity and thickening of bladder wall (*arrow*). Contrast is seen in the urethra as the patient could not retain urine.

◀──

Radiation changes within the bladder are best assessed at cystoscopy. Mucosal lesions, particularly telangiectasia, are common and cannot be assessed radiologically. Mucosal oedema and bladder wall thickening can be seen on the IVU (Fig. 3.20) and bladder wall thickness assessed by ultrasound. It is likely that abnormalities detected radiologically represent severe change. The demonstration of a bladder fistula may require radiological investigation. The majority of fistulae demonstrated in our series were vesico-vaginal defects. Cystography is a better radiological method of demonstrating these fistulae than the IVU. This is especially true for a small fistula. Associated peri-vesical fibrosis may cause alteration in bladder size and shape. The bladder may become shrunken and indistensible, changes which may be reflected on the IVU (Fig. 3.21).

Another radiological feature associated with vesical radiation disease is the presence of calcification within the bladder. It is recognised that the most likely cause of calcification is an ulcerated area becoming encrusted with urine salts due to chronic infection by urea-splitting organisms (Watson et al 1947; Maier 1972).

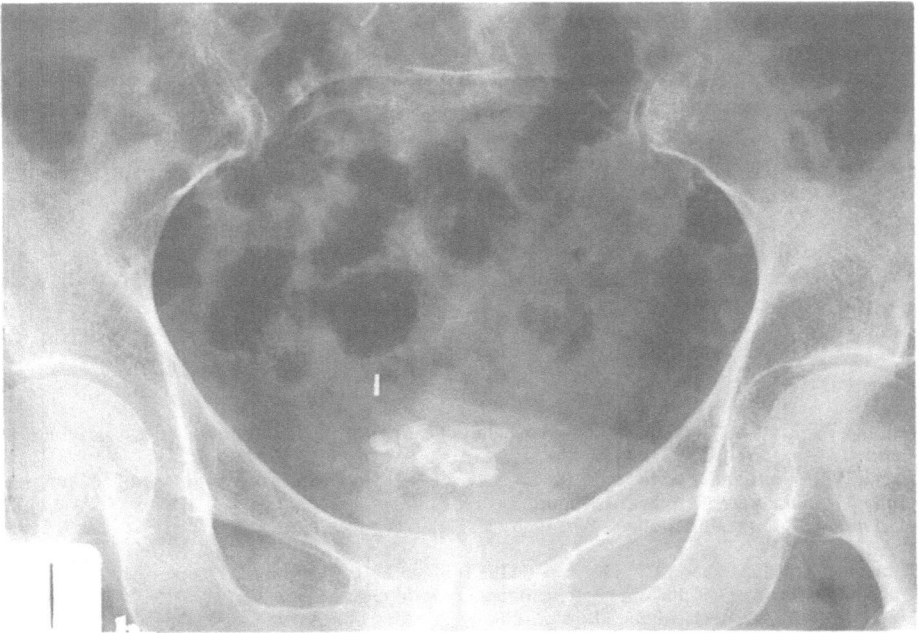

Fig. 3.21. Control radiograph for an IVU demonstrating multiple calcific opacities within the bladder. The inert seed is in the vaginal fornix.

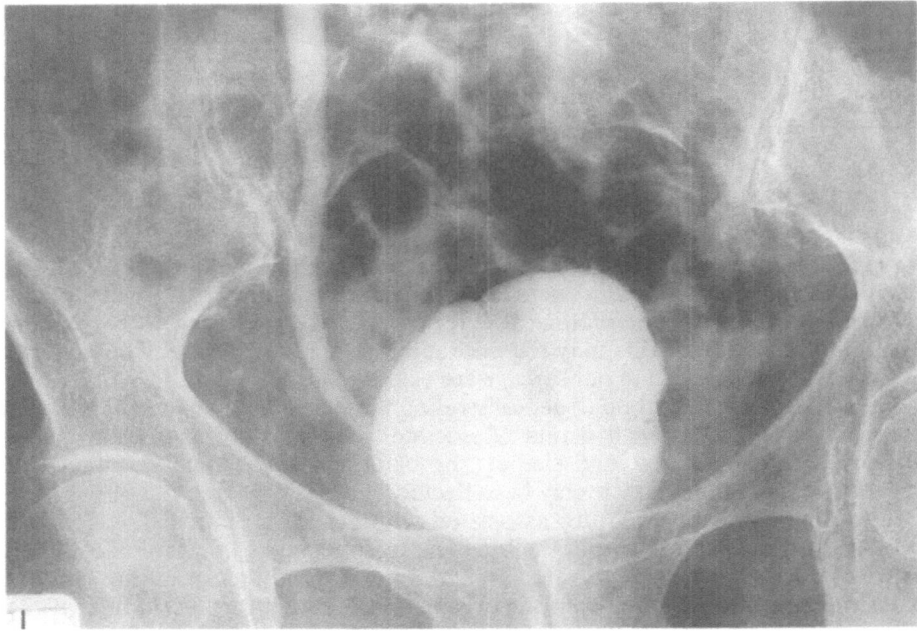

Fig. 3.22. IVU showing contrast within a small, contracted and distorted bladder. The right ureter is also dilated.

Green (1979) has reported an increased incidence of bladder calculi in necrotic areas. An example of vesical calcification after radiotherapy is shown in Fig. 3.22.

The radiological input to the problems of radiation-induced disease of the bowel and urinary tract extends from the interpretation of conventional radiography through more complex evaluations of the pelvis to some interventional procedures. The radiologist therefore has an important role in the team management of radiation disease.

References

Grainger RG (1984) The clinical and financial implications of the low-osmolar radiological contrast media. Clin Radiol 35:251–252

Green B (1979) Bladder and ureter. In: Libshitz MI (ed) Diagnostic roentgenology of radiotherapy change. Williams & Wilkins, Baltimore, pp 123–136

Hasleton PS, Carr N, Schofield PF (1985) Vascular changes in radiation bowel disease. Histopathology 9:517–534

Kjorstad KE, Martimbeau PW, Iversen T (1983) Stage 1B carcinoma of the cervix, the Norwegian Radium Hospital: results and complications. Gynecol Oncol 15:42–47

Maier JG (1972) Effects of radiation on kidney, bladder and prostate. Front Radiat Ther Oncol 6:196–227

Mason GR, Dietrich P, Friedland GW, Hanks GE (1970) The radiological findings in radiation-induced enteritis and colitis. Clin Radiol 21:232–247

Mendelson RM, Nolan DJ (1985) The radiological features of chronic radiation enteritis. Clin Radiol 36:141–148

Miller RE, Sellink JL (1979) Enteroclysis: the small bowel enema. How to succeed and how to fail. Gastrointest Radiol 4:269–283

Muram D, Oxorn M, Curry P, Walters JM (1981) Post radiation ureteral obstruction. A reappraisal. Am J Obstet Gynecol 139:289–293

Nolan DJ (1983) Radiological investigation of the small intestine. In: Whitehouse GH, Worthington B (eds) Techniques in diagnostic radiology. Blackwell Scientific Publications, Oxford, pp 21–31

O'Reilly PH, Shields RA, Testa HJ (1986) In: Nuclear medicine in urology and nephrology. Butterworths, London Boston, p 255

Rogers LF, Goldstein HM (1977) Roentgen manifestations of radiation injury to the gastrointestinal tract. Gastrointest Radiol 2:281–291

Schenker B (1964) Drip infusion pyelography. Radiology 83:12–21

Slater JM, Fletcher GH (1971) Ureteral strictures after radiation therapy for carcinoma of the uterine cervix. Am J Roentgenol 111:269–272

Walsh HPJ, Schofield PF (1984) "Is laparotomy for small bowel obstruction justified in patients with previously treated malignancy?" Br J Surg 71:933–935

Watson EM, Herger CC, Sauer HR (1947) Irradiation reactions in the bladder; their occurrence and clinical course following the use of X-ray and radium in the treatment of female pelvic disease. J Urol 57:1038–1049

Weinstein BJ, Skolnick ML (1978) Ultrasonically guided antegrade pyelography. J Urol 120:323–327

Yuhasz M, Laufer I, Sutton G, Herlinger H, Caroline DF (1985) Radiography of the small bowel in patients with gynecologic malignancies. Am J Roentgenol 144:303–307

Part 2
Bowel Disorders

4. Clinical Features of Radiation Bowel Disease

P. F. Schofield

Introduction

Radiation therapy has been used for many years to treat abdominal conditions, particularly gynaecological or urological malignancy in the pelvis. Whilst the tumour itself receives the planned dosage, it is inevitable that the adjacent bowel receives some irradiation. It is probable that subclinical bowel damage is common but good radiotherapy technique makes significant injury relatively rare (Rubin 1984).

The development of radiation bowel disease (RBD) after pelvic radiotherapy for carcinoma cervix has been variously reported as ranging from 1% to 20% of patients treated (Kjorstad et al. 1983). An increased incidence is apparent in recent years from published reports (Editorial 1984) and in our centre (Sherrah-Davies 1985).

There are three distinct time periods at which gastrointestinal problems may affect the patient: immediate (at or shortly after the radiotherapy), late (after some months) and remote (many years later) (Schofield et al. 1983). See Table 4.1. The pathological mechanisms underlying these disturbances differ. The immediate reaction is not well understood but it appears likely that the therapy affects rapidly dividing cells to induce cellular necrosis (Berthrong 1986). The late and remote effects are now well recognised as being due to ischaemia (Hasleton et al. 1985).

The site of injury depends on the radiotherapy techniques and the region irradiated. The oesophagus may be affected by techniques designed to treat

Table 4.1. Types of radiation disease

Early effects	Reaction during treatment and immediately after
Late effects	Several months later
Remote effects	Many years later

carcinoma bronchus (Lepke and Libshitz 1983), the stomach or duodenum by techniques designed to treat lymphoma (Gallez-Marchal et al. 1984) and the small bowel may react to abdominal treatment for a variety of conditions.

However, the common, important longer-term effects are related to pelvic radiotherapy (Schofield et al. 1983). The rectum and sigmoid colon are the commonest sites of injury which usually follows radiotherapy for carcinoma cervix or carcinoma bladder but we are now beginning to see cases consequent upon treatment of carcinoma prostate (Gree et al. 1984) and carcinoma rectum (Danjoux and Catton 1979). Pre-operative radiotherapy in carcinoma rectum is not associated with increased morbidity but several studies of post-operative radiotherapy have shown a significant increase in RBD (Zucali et al. 1987). Radiotherapy-related morbidity requiring re-operation is reported in up to 11% of cases receiving post-operative radiotherapy for carcinoma rectum (Gaze 1988).

Immediate Reactions

Some immediate reaction to pelvic radiotherapy is almost invariable but it is usually a relatively mild rectal reaction towards the end and shortly after the course of treatment, which settles spontaneously. Occasionally, after pelvic radiotherapy, or more often after abdominal treatment, there is a transient enteritis with diarrhoea and abdominal colic. This is usually short-lived and requires only simple treatment (Smith and DeCosse 1986). Very rarely, the diarrhoea becomes a significant problem when the patient presents with signs of peritoneal irritation or septicaemia. Perforative bowel disease is extremely unusual at this time but may occur if the patient has been on chemotherapy (Danjoux and Catton 1979). Other causes of peritoneal irritation may occur at this time. Recrudescence of previously quiescent diverticular disease or inflammatory bowel disease has been reported and should be considered if there is an appropriate history (Schofield et al. 1983). Alternatively, there may be peritonitis due to an exacerbation of gynaecological inflammatory disease. We have seen cases of tubo-ovarian abscess and pyometra developing at this stage. Finally, one should consider unrelated causes of peritonitis e.g. we have seen coincident acute appendicitis.

Late Radiation Disease

Problems which occur months or years after radiotherapy are diagnostically more challenging. Here we have the possibility of any problem being due to recurrent tumour, RBD, or a third, unrelated cause. None of these possibilities should be ignored. It has been correctly stressed that it must not be assumed that problems some months after radiotherapy are due to recurrence of tumour (Jackson 1976). Some symptoms are due to tumour but more are due to RBD. A number of patients have both processes and a few have neither as a cause of the symptoms.

It may be stating the obvious that one has to think of a diagnosis before one can make it. However, this is pertinent in bowel disease which develops late after radiotherapy. The longer the time gap between radiotherapy and symptoms of bowel disease the more likely it is for the significance of preceding therapy to be overlooked. Many of the patients with RBD referred to us had other diagnoses made by experienced clinicians. Although the cause ultimately proved to be RBD we have had patients referred with rectal bleeding with a diagnosis of haemorrhoids, with bloody diarrhoea referred as non-specific inflammatory bowel disease, with peri-colic abscesses referred as diverticular disease. Perhaps of even greater significance is the misdiagnosis of recurrent, incurable malignancy. This leads to mismanagement and prevents prompt referral.

Predisposing Factors

It is important to recognise factors which may predispose to RBD. It is clear that radiation to the pelvis is particularly likely to be complicated by RBD and the factors relating to technique have been fully discussed in Chapter 1. From the gastrointestinal point of view, it is important to realise that therapy by single modalities, whether by external beam or intracavity techniques tend to produce more localised lesions than when both modalities are used (Carr et al. 1984).

The tolerance of normal tissues to radiotherapy can be altered by a number of factors as well as those associated with the radiotherapy technique. There seems little doubt that related chemotherapy increases the susceptibility to damage (Danjoux and Catton 1979) as does previous pelvic surgery (DeCosse et al. 1969). Pre-existing conditions have been shown to "sensitise" the patient. These conditions include diabetes mellitus, hypertension and arteriosclerosis (DeCosse et al. 1969). All of these are linked by a tendency to vascular narrowing so that the reduced vascular volume characteristic of late radiation change is more likely to produce clinical manifestations. Whether a severe early reaction predisposes a patient to the development of late radiation disease is still in dispute. The relationship is denied by many authors but a recent study has shown that later development of radiation disease is three times more likely in patients who have had a severe early reaction (Bourne et al. 1983).

Conversely, previous pelvic radiotherapy constitutes a major risk factor after surgery to the abdominal aorta. Rectal necrosis has been reported after aortic bifurcation graft in patients who had pelvic radiotherapy many years previously (Harling et al. 1986).

Clinical Presentation

It is convenient to discuss the clinical problems presented in late radiation disease according to their principal presenting symptom (Table 4.2). Between 6 months and 2 years after treatment there are five types of presentation: rectal bleeding, intestinal obstruction, chronic perforation with abscess, anal or perineal pain and recto-vaginal fistula.

Rectal Bleeding. Although this is the commonest, it is the least serious of the five types of presentation. Many of the patients have relatively minor bleeding but a

Table 4.2. Timing relation of various presentations

Presentation	Time between XRT and onset
Acute proctitis	0–1 month
Rectal bleeding	4–12 months
Acute enteritis	0–1 month
Chronic abscess	9–15 months
Anal/perineal pain	6–9 months
Fistula	1.5–2 years
Stricture ± malabsorption	2–20 years
Rectal malignancy	5–40 years

few have more significant blood loss which requires repeated blood transfusion. Gilinsky et al. (1983) surveyed this aspect. They found that most patients with minor bleeding settled spontaneously within 18 months but if the bleeding was severe enough to require blood transfusion or was associated with abdominal pain then surgery was frequently required. Diagnosis is usually straightforward as there are typical findings of radiation proctitis within easy reach of the sigmoidoscope. Occasionally, the affected area is in the sigmoid colon and requires a flexible endoscope to reach the abnormality. Sometimes a misdiagnosis of non-specific ulcerative procto-colitis can be made by the unwary because of failure to recognise the significance of previous radiotherapy.

Intestinal Obstruction. Symptoms of low small bowel obstruction are a common method of presentation of patients with ileal radiation disease. Early incomplete obstruction can pose diagnostic difficulties. The patient may give a history of abdominal colic after food with some distension but both physical and radiological examinations yield no abnormal findings. Detailed small bowel contrast studies may indicate the lesion but are not absolutely reliable and tend to underestimate the severity of the problem.

It is usual for this type of patient to progress and may present after a series of minor attacks with more manifest obstruction. At this stage, the patient has more persistent abdominal colic and vomiting with abdominal distension. The obstruction is usually incomplete so that there is rarely absolute constipation but plain radiographs of the abdomen show multiple small bowel distended loops with fluid levels. When patients have had previous radiotherapy, experience would indicate that RBD is a commoner cause of small bowel obstruction than recurrent tumour or other unrelated causes (Walsh and Schofield 1984). Abdominal examination may show distension and tenderness in the right lower quadrant or there may be tenderness in the pelvis on rectal examination. A mass may be appreciated in the area of tenderness especially if examination under anaesthesia is carried out.

Chronic Perforation with Abscess. Due to the slow development of ischaemia, there may be a necrotic area of the bowel wall which has been sealed off by the surrounding tissues. This process leads to localised sepsis – a chronic perforation with abscess. When the large bowel is involved by this process, the patient may have some colic and possibly some distension of the large bowel but the symptoms of sepsis predominate over those of intestinal obstruction. In this type of presentation, the patient has disturbance of bowel function with abdominal pain. Examination may show distension and a mass may be present either on abdominal or rectal examination. This is the type of case in which it is all too easy for the clinician to believe that there is recurrent, disseminated abdominal malignancy. It may be difficult to distinguish recurrent malignancy from RBD before operation despite sophisticated examination and, on occasions, both recurrence and RBD co-exist. It is accepted as an aphorism in our clinic that this type of case is due to radiation until proved otherwise.

From the practical point of view, all these cases require operation which may be curative in the patients with RBD and can often effect good palliation in the patient with recurrent malignancy.

Anal or Perineal Pain. Ulceration in the anal canal may occur and cause pain. The pain may occur only at defaecation but in other patients it is a persistent severe perineal discomfort (Schofield et al. 1983). In our experience, this problem occurs within a few months of treatment. The condition is seen most frequently after radiotherapy for carcinoma prostate but it can occur after therapy for carcinoma cervix. Although minor ulceration may heal, the patients frequently come to radical excisional surgery as the only method of pain relief. In the female, there is a risk of a persistent ulcer progressing to form a fistula to the vagina after a few months. It is important to avoid biopsy of the ulcer as this may precipitate the fistula.

Fistula. A fistula to the vagina may involve the gastrointestinal or urinary tract. The commonest type seen after radiation is a recto-vaginal fistula (Smith and DeCosse 1986) leading to faecal "incontinence" and general perineal discomfort. There is usually little difficulty in confirming the diagnosis at examination but the patient may be so swollen and sore that examination is difficult. When the recto-vaginal fistula is fully established it is necessary to know whether this fistula is due to recurrent tumour or due to pure radiation change and at this stage biopsy is safe and necessary. In most patients examination under anaesthesia is useful to allow adequate assessment and biopsy.

Investigation of Late Radiation Bowel Disease

Awareness of the possibility of the diagnosis, and clinical assessment of the patient are of paramount importance. Investigations can help in resolving certain problems and are directed towards:

1. The general state of the patient
2. The differentiation between recurrent tumour and radiation change
3. The accurate localisation of the radiation change.

General Assessment. Many of these patients are anaemic and have various degrees of malnutrition. For this reason, full haematological and biochemical assessment is desirable. In addition, such other investigations are carried out as may be indicated by the clinical state of the patient to assess the general condition.

RBD versus Recurrence. The distinction can be very difficult. A chest x-ray is mandatory to exclude pulmonary metastases and in many instances ultrasonography or a radionuclide scan of the liver is used to exclude metastases at this site. We have found that the platelet count is frequently elevated in active RBD and this may be helpful in differentiation (Carr et al. 1985). Ideally, a tissue diagnosis by biopsy is desirable but frequently this is impractical before surgery.

Localisation of Disease. For this we are dependent upon endoscopy (sigmoidoscopy and/or colonoscopy) and radiological imaging techniques, which are fully discussed in Chapter 3. Because of the frequent occurrence of RBD and urinary tract injury in the same patient we would advocate an assessment of the urinary tract in patients with RBD when the clinical situation allows it (Schofield et al. 1986).

Remote Radiation Disease

Many years after radiotherapy, the patients may present with symptoms of incomplete ileal or colonic obstruction or with a malabsorption syndrome. This situation requires great vigilance because the radiotherapy was so long ago that the patient will rarely associate the problem.

Intestinal Obstruction

Symptoms in patients presenting with intestinal obstruction vary with the anatomical site of the obstructing lesion. Patients with an ileal stricture present with colic and distension but there is usually a history of vomiting and diarrhoea. Plain radiography will confirm low small bowel obstruction and the provisional diagnosis is usually made, provided the significance of previous irradiation is understood. These patients rarely have a mass or associated sepsis as the lesion is an ischaemic stricture of variable length. Similarly, patients with a colo-rectal stricture present with typical features of incomplete large bowel obstruction. In our experience, these late strictures are usually situated in the sigmoid colon.

Malabsorption

Diarrhoea is the commonest clinical manifestation of chronic, non-obstructive ileal disease but it may also be seen after small bowel resection or in association with an ileal stricture. There are several potential mechanisms underlying the diarrhoea – it may be due to a lessening of the absorptive capacity of the small bowel after resection, it may be due to defective bile salt absorption in the damaged terminal ileum so that the bile acids irritate the colon or it may be due to small bowel bacterial colonisation above a stricture (Ludgate and Merrick 1985). Ileal resection or disease may lead to defective absorption of vitamin B12 leading to megaloblastic anaemia. Associated features of malnutrition may include hypocalcaemia and hypoproteinaemia. If the stool is assessed for fat, the patients will frequently be found to have steatorrhoea.

These conditions can be elucidated by adequate investigation. Full haematological and biochemical assessment is indicated. ^{75}Se-homocholic acid taurine (SeHCAT) is a radio-labelled, synthetic bile acid which, when taken by mouth, enables the detection of defective bile acid absorption by whole body scanning (Ludgate and Merrick 1985). Small bowel colonisation can be demonstrated by breath hydrogen estimation (Rhodes et al. 1979). Other specialised tests may be indicated for specific individual problems.

Association with Rectal Carcinoma

Malignant change in the gastrointestinal tract may occur in areas which have been in a therapeutic radiation field (Berthrong 1986). In an individual patient it is difficult to be certain whether any malignancy which develops is induced by the radiation or is coincidental. This difficulty is enhanced by the fact that malignant change occurs many years after the radiation treatment. Several examples seem to follow relatively low dosage treatment, such as the development of upper oesophageal carcinoma after radiotherapy for thyrotoxicosis and the occurrence of pelvic cancer after low dosage treatment to induce an artificial menopause (Berthrong 1986). There is an excess mortality due to carcinoma colon in the survivors of the Hiroshima and Nagasaki atomic bomb explosions (Kato and Schull 1982). These patients probably had a dose of radiation in excess of therapeutic levels.

It seems possible that carcinoma of the rectum may be induced many years after high-dose therapeutic radiation to the pelvis (Sandler and Sandler 1983). There are several reports from the literature that suggest this is a true relationship (Black and Ackerman 1965) and we have seen a number of cases of rectal carcinoma which presented many years after radiotherapy treatment for either carcinoma cervix or carcinoma bladder. A recent report reviews 76 cases of carcinoma of the colon or rectum developing many years after pelvic radiotherapy for other conditions. The mean interval between radiation and the development of the cancer was 15.2 years (Shu-Wen Jao et al. 1987). Sandler and Sandler (1983) suggest that the risk of developing carcinoma rectum in females who have received pelvic radiotherapy for cancer is somewhere between two and four times that of the normal population.

References

Berthrong M (1986) Pathologic changes secondary to radiation. World J Surg 10:155–170

Black WC, Ackerman LV (1965) Carcinoma of the large intestine as a late complication of pelvic radiotherapy. Clin Radiol 16:278–281

Bourne RG, Kearsley JH, Grove WD, Roberts SJ (1983) The relationship between early and late gastrointestinal complications of radiation therapy for carcinoma of the cervix. Int J Radiat Oncol Biol Phys 9:1445–1450

Carr ND, Pullen BR, Hasleton PS, Schofield PF (1984) Microvascular studies in human radiation bowel disease. Gut 25:448–454

Carr ND, Hasleton PS, Schofield PF (1985) Platelet count in radiation bowel disease: An aid to diagnosis. Br J Surg 72:287–288

Danjoux CE, Catton GE (1979) Delayed complications in colorectal carcinoma treated by combination radiotherapy and 5-fluorouracil – Eastern Cooperative (ECOG) Pilot Study. Int J Radiat Oncol Biol Phys 5:311–316

DeCosse JJ, Rhodes RS, Wentz WB, Reagan JW, Dworken HJ, Holden WD (1969) The natural history and management of radiation induced injury of the gastrointestinal tract. Ann Surg 170:369–384

Editorial (1984) Radiation bowel disease. Lancet ii:963–964

Gallez-Marchal D, Foyolle M, Henry-Amar M, Le Bourgeois JP, Rougier P, Cosset JM (1984) Radiation injuries of the gastrointestinal tract in Hodgkin's disease. Radiotherapy and Oncology 2:93–99

Gaze MN (1988) Review: radiotherapy for rectal carcinoma. J R Coll Surg Edin 33:175–178

Gilinsky NH, Burns DG, Barbezat GO, Levin W, Myers HS, Marks IN (1983) The natural history of radiation induced proctosigmoiditis: analysis of 88 patients. Q J Med 52:40–53

Gree N, Goldman H, Lombardo L, Skaist L (1984) Severe rectal injury following radiation for prostatic cancer. J Urol 131:701–704

Harling H, Balslev I, Larsen JF (1986) Necrosis of the rectum complicating abdominal aortic reconstructions in previously irradiated patients. Br J Surg 73:711

Hasleton PS, Carr ND, Schofield PF (1985) Vascular changes in radiation bowel disease. Histopathology 9:517–534

Jackson BT (1976) Bowel damage from radiation. Proc R Soc Med 69:683–686

Kato H, Schull WJ (1982) Studies of the mortality of A-bomb survivors, 1950–1978. I. Cancer mortality. Radiat Res 90:395–432

Kjorstad KE, Martimbeau PW, Iversen T (1983) Stage 1B carcinoma of the cervix, the Norwegian Radium Hospital: results and complications. Gynecol Oncol 15:42–47

Lepke RA, Libshitz HI (1983) Radiation-induced injury of the oesophagus. Radiology 148:375–378

Ludgate SM, Merrick MV (1985) The pathogenesis of post-irradiation chronic diarrhoea: measurement of SeHCAT and B12 absorption for differential diagnosis determines treatment. Clin Radiol 36:275–278

Rhodes JM, Middleton P, Jewell DP (1979) The lactulose hydrogen breath test as a diagnostic test for small-bowel bacterial overgrowth. Scand J Gastroenterol 14:333–336

Rubin P (1984) Late effects of chemotherapy and radiation therapy: a new hypothesis. Int J Radiat Oncol Biol Phys 10:5–34

Sandler RS, Sandler DP (1983) Radiation induced cancers of the colon and rectum. Assessing the risk. Gastroenterology 84:51–57

Schofield PF, Holden D, Carr ND (1983) Bowel disease after radiotherapy. J R Soc Med 76:463–466

Schofield PF, Carr ND, Holden D (1986) The pathogenesis and treatment of radiation bowel disease. J R Soc Med 79:30–32

Sherrah-Davies E (1985) Morbidity after selectron therapy for cervical cancer. Clin Radiol 36:131–139

Shu-Wen Jao MD, Beart RW, Reiman HM, Gunderson LL, Ilstrup DM (1987) Colon and anorectal cancer after pelvic irradiation. Dis Colon Rectum 30:953–958

Smith DH, DeCosse JJ (1986) Radiation damage to the small intestine. World J Surg 10:189–194

Walsh HPJ, Schofield PF (1984) Is laparotomy for small bowel obstruction justified in patients with previously treated malignancy? Br J Surg 71:933–935

Zucali R, Gardani G, Lattuada A (1987) Adjuvant irradiation after radical surgery of cancer of the rectum and rectosigmoid. Radiother Oncol 8:19–24

5. Experimental Findings in Radiation Bowel Disease

N. D. Carr and D. Holden

Introduction

The pathological response of the bowel to radiation is complex, but histological changes in small vessels are commonly found in radiation damaged bowel (Berthrong and Fajardo 1981). It has been postulated that these vascular lesions may compromise the microvasculature of the bowel and lead to progressive ischaemia (Ashbaugh and Owens 1963; DeCosse et al. 1969). Although there is evidence from studies in experimental animals to support this hypothesis (Eddy and Casarett 1968; Eriksson 1982) the role of small-vessel disease in the pathogenesis of human radiation bowel disease (RBD) remains unclear.

The purpose of the present chapter is twofold; first, to review the histological types of vascular injury which occur at the site of human radiation bowel disease and, second, to describe the overall effects of these lesions on the intramural vasculature in human bowel.

Histological Changes in Blood Vessels

Qualitative Vascular Changes

Several authors have drawn attention to the characteristic vascular changes which are present at the site of radiation bowel injury (Sheehan 1944; Perkins and Spjut 1962; Localio et al. 1979; Berthrong and Fajardo 1981). Lesions are present in the medium-sized muscular arteries of the distal mesentery and are most pronounced in areas adjacent to strictures and necrosis or fistulae. The most common of these is intimal fibrosis (Fig. 5.1a,b) which is of variable degree and sometimes admixed with oedema fluid and fibrin fluid (Fig. 5.2). The structural integrity of the media is usually well preserved but lesions may be apparent in some vessels. Acute inflammatory infiltration, with or without fibrinoid change, occurs in some

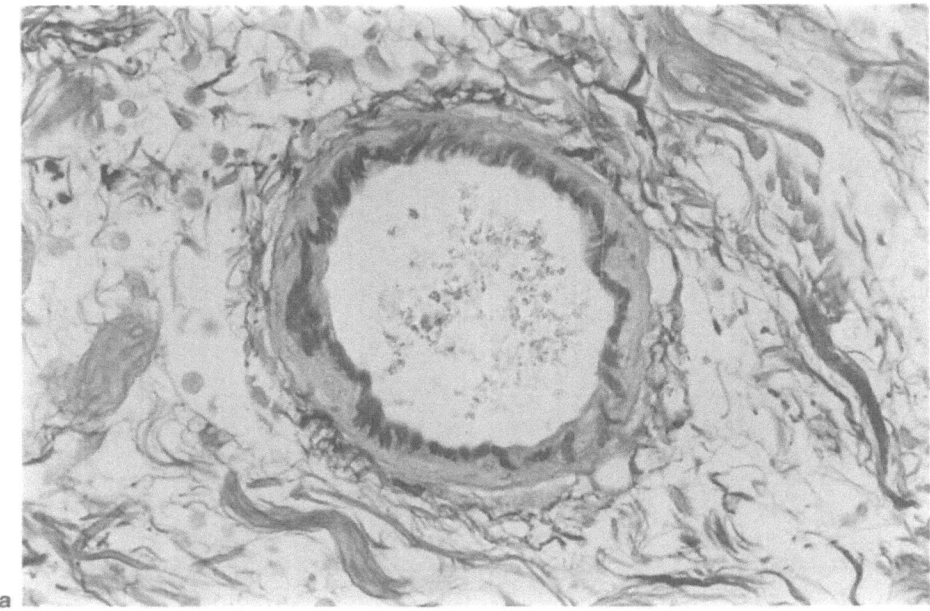

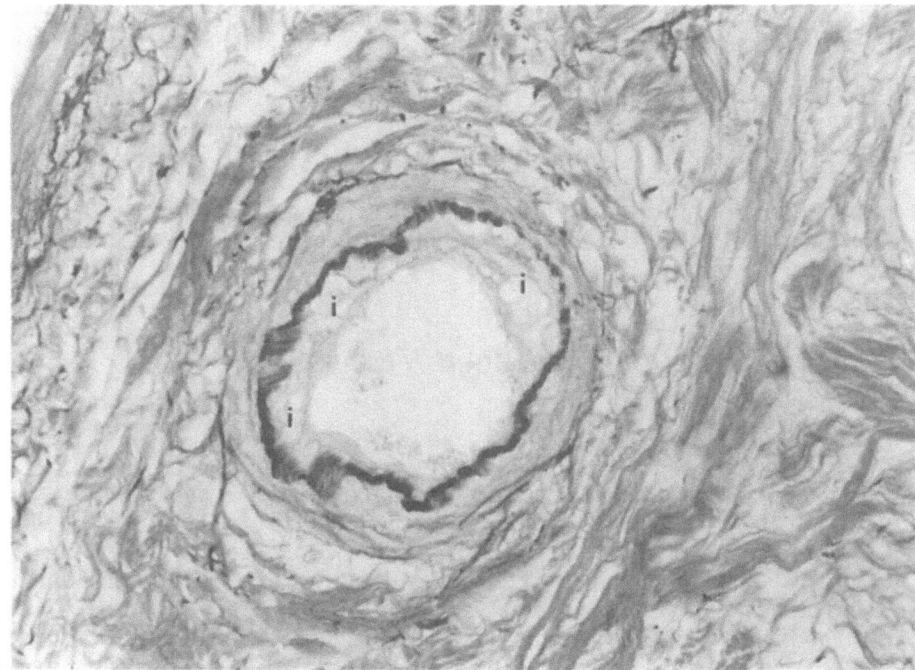

Fig. 5.1.a,b   Small mesenteric arteries from normal bowel (*top*) and from RBD (*bottom*). The latter shows intimal fibrosis (*i*). (EVG ×200)

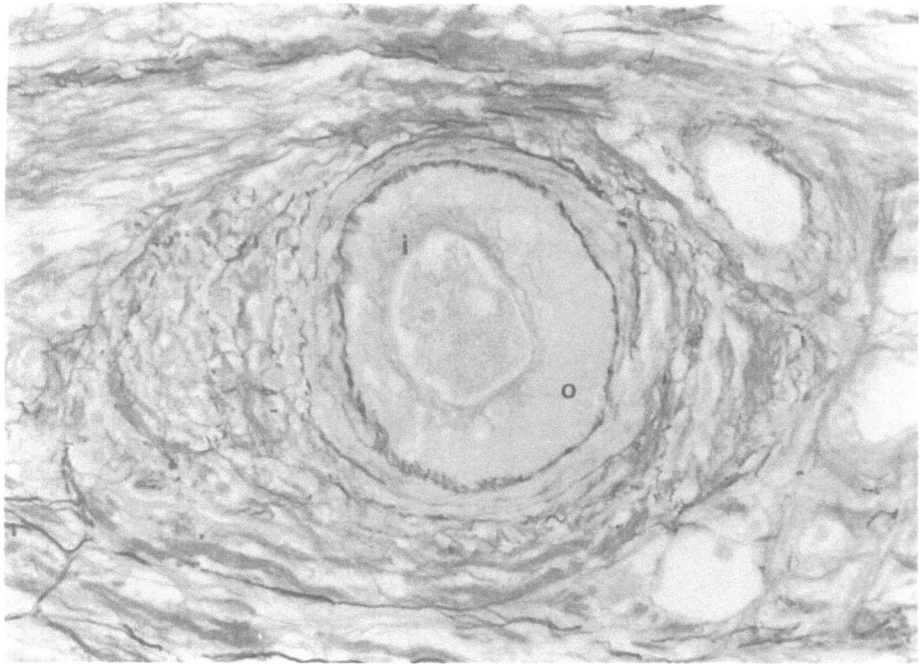

Fig. 5.2. Small mesenteric artery in RBD. Shows marked intimal thickening produced by intimal fibrosis (*i*) and oedema fluid (*o*). (EVG ×200)

muscular arteries (Fig. 5.3). In other vessels the media shows evidence of cystic degeneration which usually occurs in association with severe intimal fibrosis. These spaces can sometimes be seen to contain red blood cells and are thought to represent telangiectatic vasa vasorum (Carr et al. 1985a) (Fig. 5.4). The internal elastic lamina remains in continuity in the majority of vessels, but is often of a crenated or wrinkled configuration (Fig. 5.4), particularly in those vessels affected by severe intimal fibrosis.

Small muscular arteries and arterioles are especially vulnerable to the effects of radiation and the severe damage which may be sustained by these structures after pelvic irradiation has been examined in detail by Sheehan and others (Sheehan 1944; Perkins and Spjut 1962; Carr et al. 1985a). In the small submucosal arteries and arterioles intimal fibrosis is present in strictured areas and is often occlusive in nature (Fig. 5.5). Intimal thickening is also produced by the subendothelial deposition of oedema fluid and fibrin. In some cases these deposits of fibrin are capped with more mature fibrous tissue (Fig. 5.6). Where the bowel wall has undergone necrosis, arterioles show hyalinisation of the media, infiltration by acute and chronic inflammatory cells and fibrinoid necrosis (Fig. 5.7). Subintimal foam cells were a common feature in Sheehan's material (1944) but these cells are infrequent in the authors' experience (Carr et al. 1985a) (Fig. 5.8). Although Perkins and Spjut (1962) stressed that foam cells constitute a specific response to radiation injury, they have been observed in arteries of the non-irradiated uterus and placenta (Fajardo and Berthrong 1978). In view of these findings, it seems that these cells constitute a non-specific response to vascular injury. Berthrong

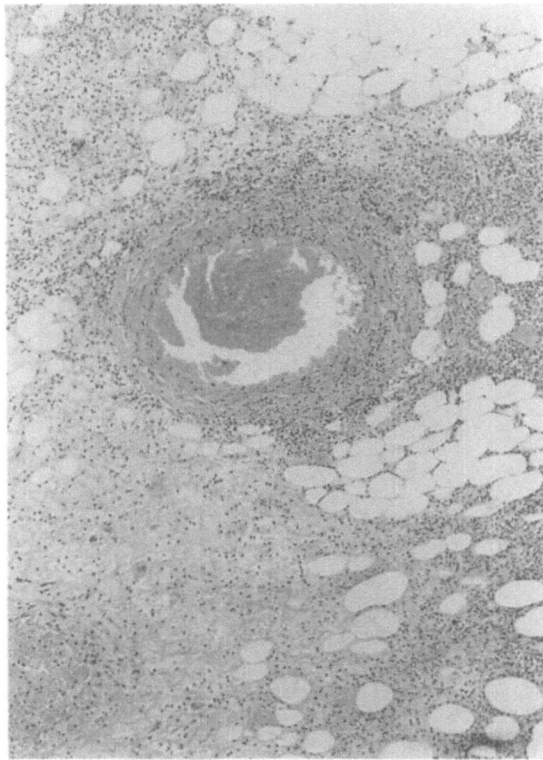

Fig. 5.3. Small mesenteric artery in RBD. Shows acute inflammatory cell infiltration of the arterial wall. (H&E ×60)

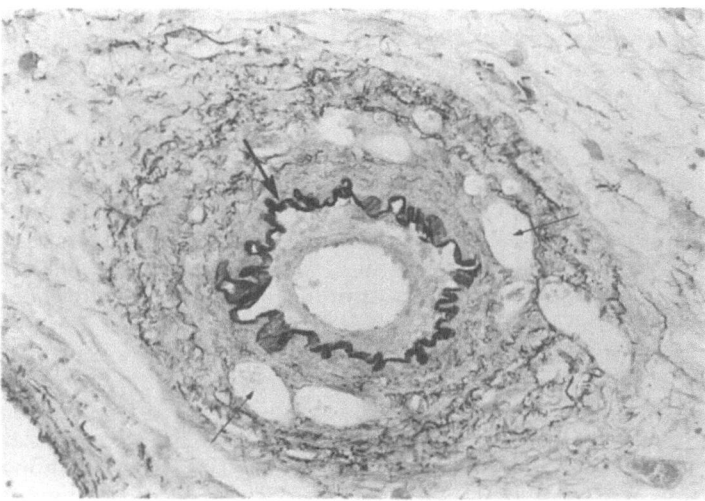

Fig. 5.4. Small mesenteric artery in RBD. The media shows numerous cystic spaces (*thin arrows*) some of which contain blood cells and represent telangiectatic vasa vasorum. The internal elastic lamina (*thick arrow*) has a crenated appearance. (EVG ×160)

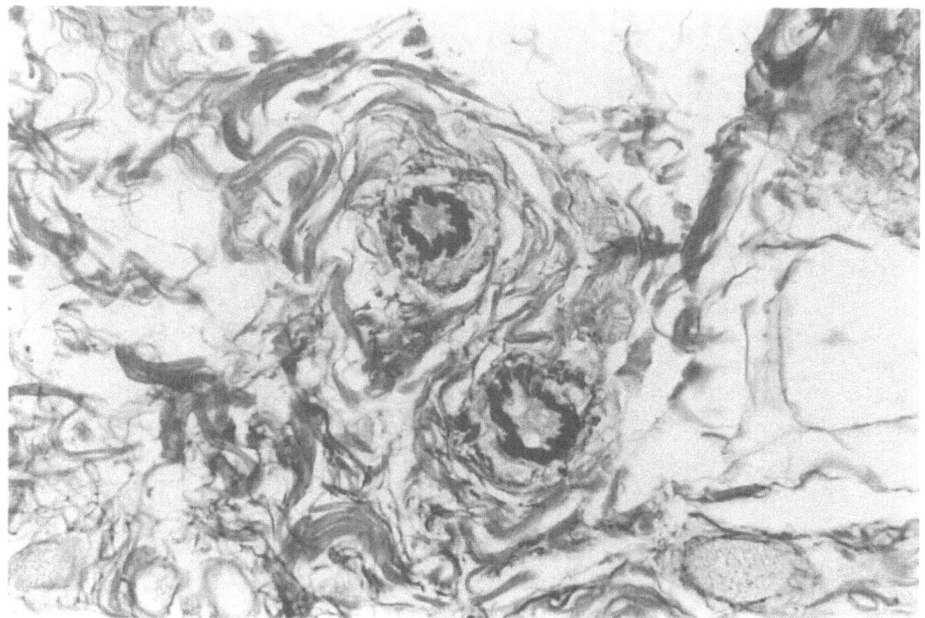

Fig. 5.5. Submucosal arterioles in RBD. Both show occlusive intimal fibrosis. (EVG ×470)

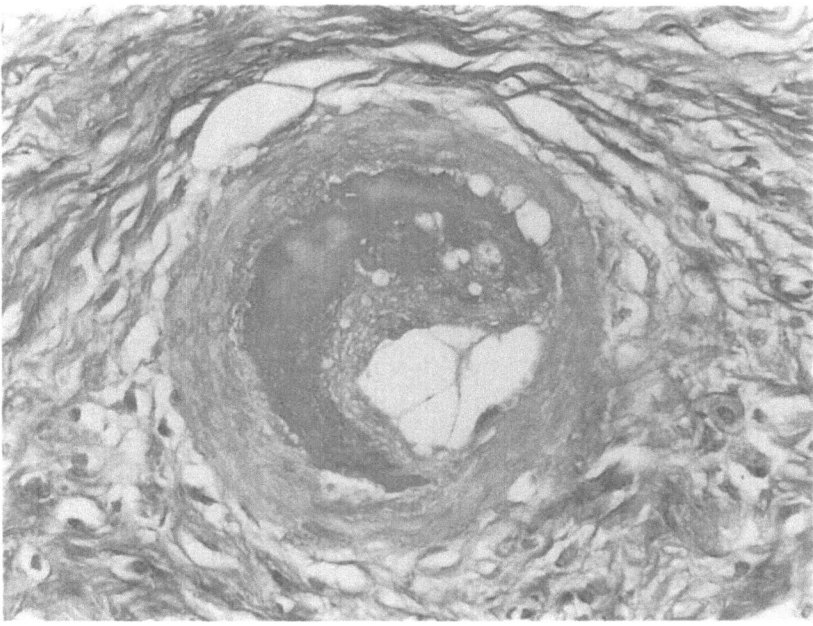

Fig. 5.6. Submucosal arteriole in RBD. Shows subendothelial deposit of fibrin covered by fibrous tissue. (MSB ×290)

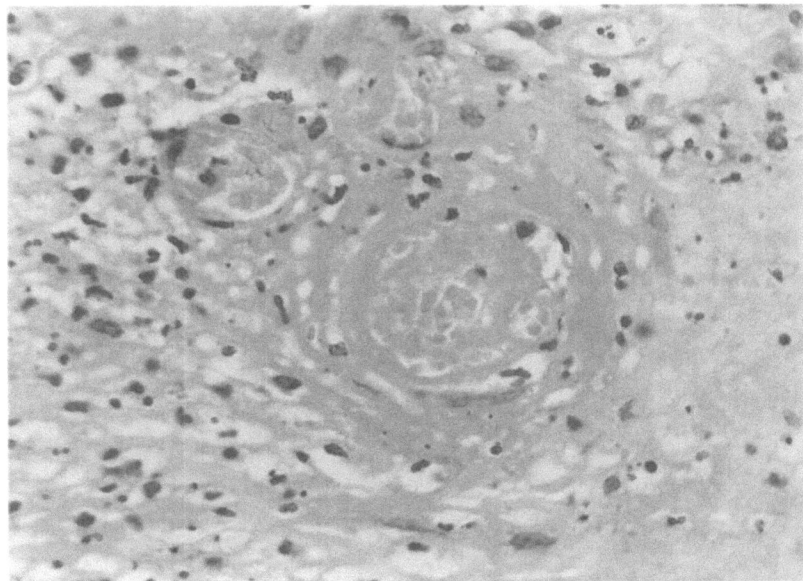

Fig. 5.7. Submucosal arteriole in RBD. There is fibrinoid necrosis of the media and in this case the lumen is occluded by fibrin thrombus. (H&E ×460)

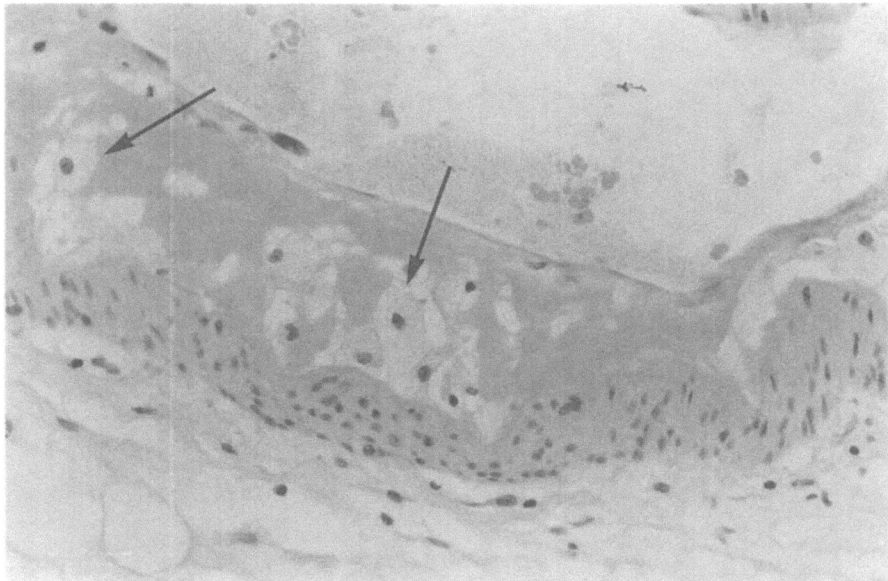

Fig. 5.8. Part of the wall of a small submucosal artery in RBD sectioned longitudinally. Shows collections of subintimal foam cells (*arrows*). These were uncommon in the authors' experience. (H&E ×290)

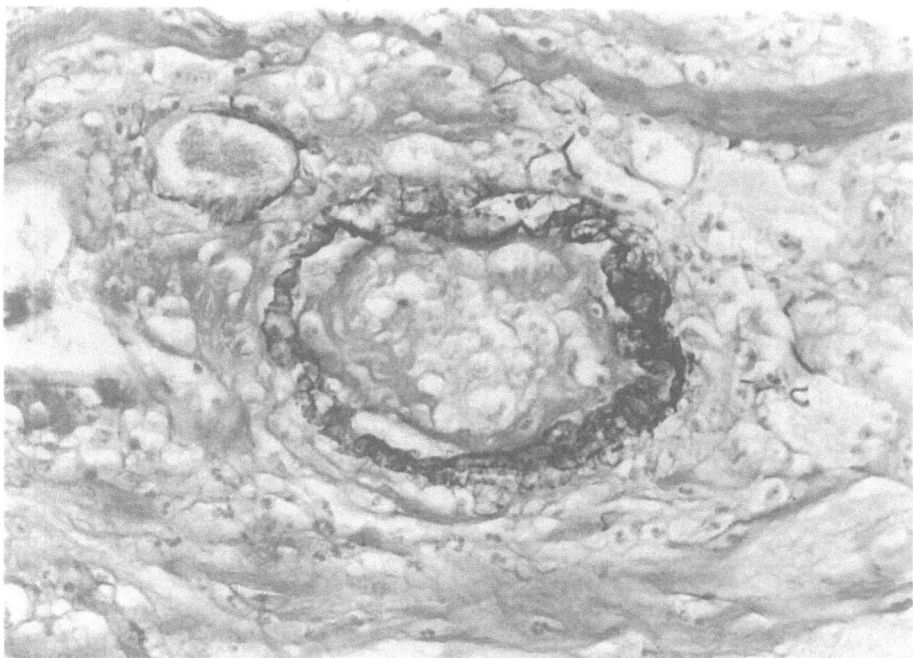

Fig. 5.9.   Submucosal venule in RBD which shows occlusive intimal fibrosis. (EVG ×320)

and Fajardo (1981) have stated that venous lesions are uncommon in association with RBD. In contrast, severe venous injury in the form of intimal fibrosis and thrombosis has been seen in other series (Carr et al. 1985a) (Fig. 5.9) and it should be emphasised that occlusive venous changes may be just as detrimental to microvascular function as arterial and arteriolar lesions.

Telangiectasia is also present. This change occurs focally in the capillaries from otherwise normal mucosa (Fig. 5.10) and bizarre and florid displays of ectatic thin-walled vessels situated amongst hyaline fibrous tissue are also seen in the submucosa (Berthrong and Fajardo 1981; Carr et al. 1985a) (Fig. 5.11).

Quantitative Vascular Changes

The authors have examined blood vessels in human RBD using vascular morphometry (Carr et al. 1985a). In this study the medial and intimal thickness of small extramural and intramural arteries (>100 μm in external diameter) and arterioles (<100 μm in external diameter) were measured using light microscopy. These indices were then expressed as a percentage of the external vessel diameter. In addition, the incidence of vessels with intimal thickening was assessed as a percentage of the total number of vessels in each specimen. Vessels from 16 patients with radiation damaged bowel and from a control group of 45 patients were examined.

The results of this study confirm that in human RBD the degree and incidence

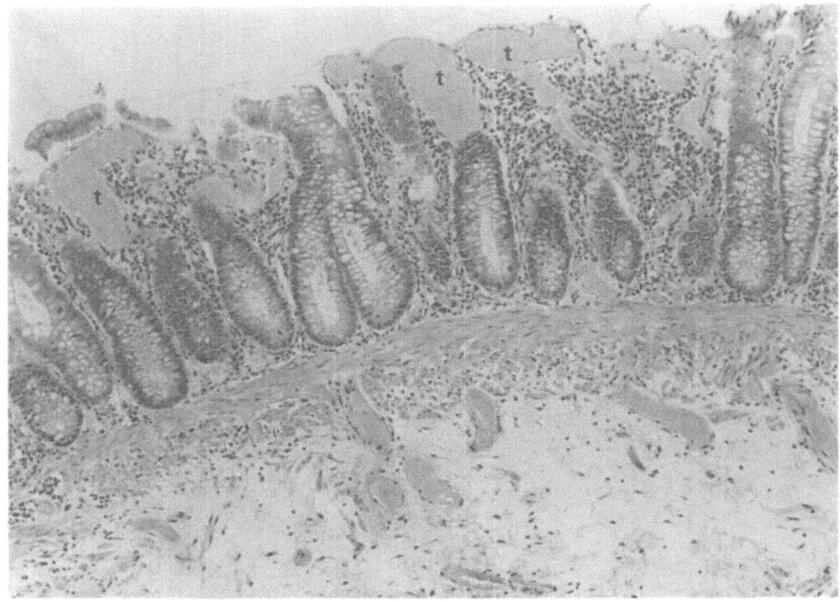

Fig. 5.10.   Mucosa from radiation disease of the sigmoid colon. Shows telangiectatic capillaries (*t*) situated in normal mucosa. (H&E ×40)

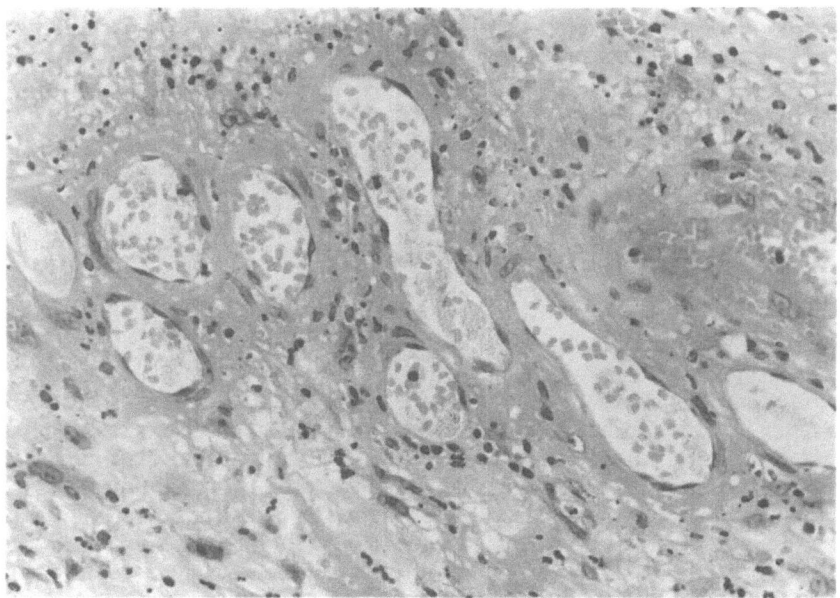

Fig. 5.11.   Submucosa from radiation disease of the sigmoid colon. Florid display of ectatic, thin-walled vessels. (H&E ×170)

of intimal thickening in small submucosal arteries and arterioles is significantly higher than that present in normal bowel (Table 5.1). The degree of intimal thickening and the incidence of intimal thickening in small arteries and arterioles is directly related to the initial dose of radiation (Table 5.2). These findings support those of others who have concluded that the magnitude of radiation-

Table 5.1. Comparison of morphometric indices between RBD and control group ($*P<0.05$)

	RBD ($n=16$)	Control ($n=45$)
Extramural vessels		
<100 μm		
Medial thickness	11.8 ± 2.2%	8.8 ± 1.3%*
Intimal thickness	6.7 ± 3.0%	5.2 ± 2.2%
No. of measured arterioles with intimal thickening	43.0 ± 24.9%	7.2 ± 9.7%*
>100 μm		
Medial thickness	11.5 ± 2.4%	8.9 ± 1.9%*
Intimal thickness	6.6 ± 3.2%	4.1 ± 2.0%
No. of measured arteries with intimal thickening	47.5 ± 24.1%	33.7 ± 19.4%
Intramural vessels		
<100 μm		
Medial thickness	10.5 ± 1.2%	8.7 ± 1.5%*
Intimal thickness	8.3 ± 2.4%	5.9 ± 1.9%*
No. of measured arterioles with intimal thickening	50.9 ± 25.9%	15.0 ± 12.4%*
>100 μm		
Medial thickness	9.6 ± 1.3%	7.7 ± 1.7%*
Intimal thickness	9.3 ± 6.2%	4.0 ± 2.6%*
No. of measured arteries with intimal thickening	51.4 ± 29.5%	16.7 ± 14.7%*

Table 5.2. Correlations in RBD ($n=16$). $*=P<0.05$

	Radiation dose	Time interval between administration of radiotherapy and onset of bowel symptoms
Extramural vessels		
<100 μm		
Medial thickness		
Intimal thickness	*	
No. of measured arterioles with intimal thickening	*	
>100 μm		
Medial thickness		*
Intimal thickness		
No. of measured arteries with intimal thickening		*
Intramural vessels		
<100 μm		
Medial thickness		
Intimal thickness	*	
No. of measured arterioles with intimal thickening	*	
>100 μm		
Medial thickness		*
Intimal thickness		*
No. of measured arteries with intimal thickening	*	

induced vascular injury is dose dependent (Eddy and Casarett 1968; Bosniak et al. 1969; Eriksson 1982). Furthermore small arteries and arterioles from radiation damaged bowel exhibited medial hypertrophy (Table 5.1) which was seen in the absence of significant systemic hypertension (Carr et al. 1985a). It seems likely that this change has occurred as a compensatory response to the increased resistance to blood flow induced by obliteration of the microvascular bed by intimal fibrosis and fibrin thrombi.

Fibrin Thrombi and Injury to Vascular Endothelium

Fibrin thrombi are present in the lumina of small arteries, arterioles (Fig. 5.7) and capillaries. These are most frequently seen in areas of necrosis (Fig. 5.12) but are also present in capillaries of intact mucosa (Carr et al. 1985a) (Fig. 5.13). It is of interest that microthrombosis of the gastrointestinal tract mucosa is a prominent feature of other colonic diseases which are presumed to have an ischaemic basis, such as necrotising enterocolitis (Ming and Levitan 1960; McGovern and Goulston 1965), and pseudomembranous colitis (Bogomoletz 1976). In these conditions and in RBD, the presence of fibrin thrombi in the capillaries of intact mucosa indicates that these lesions may be important in the pathogenesis of mucosal necrosis, but the precise stimulus for their initial formation remains uncertain. Whitehead (1971) and Margaretten and McKay (1971) believe that thrombosis of the intestinal microcirculation is a manifestation of the disseminated intravascular coagulation syndrome. It is unlikely that this is a cause of microvascular thrombosis in RBD in view of the lack of any clinical evidence of consumptive coagulopathy and the increased platelet count which has been observed in patients with radiation bowel disease (Carr et al. 1985b). Furthermore, the area of bowel involved in RBD is less extensive than that in pseudomembranous or necrotising enterocolitis, which suggests a local source of injury as a cause of microvascular thrombosis. It is probable that fibrin thrombi form in capillaries and arterioles whose endothelium has been damaged by irradiation. This hypothesis gains support from an electron microscopic study by Fajardo and Stewart (1973) of irradiated rabbit myocardium. These authors described injury to capillary endothelial cells in the form of luminal projections of cytoplasm, focal cytoplasmic thinning or bleb formation and cell necrosis which occurred immediately after exposure, reached their peak at day 20, and persisted until about 50 days. Thereafter, these acute changes progressively declined but were still present 134 days after irradiation. During the peak period of injury, obstruction to the lumen of damaged capillaries was produced by swollen endothelial cells and fibrin-platelet thrombi. In addition, these authors found a decrease in the number of capillaries which were replaced by vesicular structures bounded by remnants of endothelial cells. The presence of fibrin thrombi in RBD indicates that injury to microvascular endothelium is an important factor in human radiation bowel disease.

Acute injury to the endothelium of large arteries may occur soon after irradiation. In a scanning and transmission electron microscopic study of irradiated femoral arteries in dogs, Fonkalsrud et al. (1977) demonstrated destruction of the endothelial surface and cell necrosis 48 hours after exposure. This acute change was followed by the regeneration of an endothelial surface which was irregular and abnormal 4 months after irradiation. Taken in conjunc-

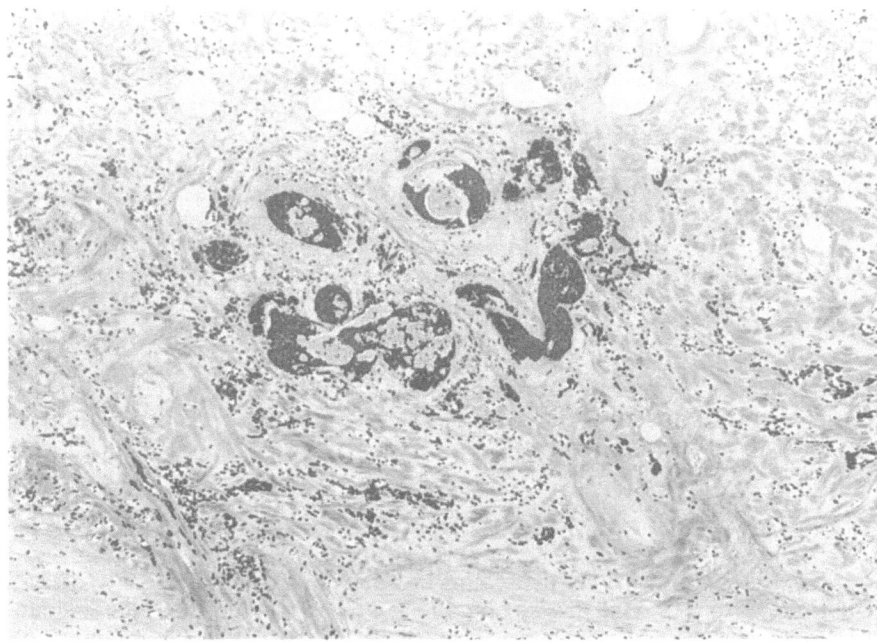

Fig. 5.12. Photomicrograph showing fibrin thrombi in vessels from an area of necrotic muscularis propria. (PTAH ×80)

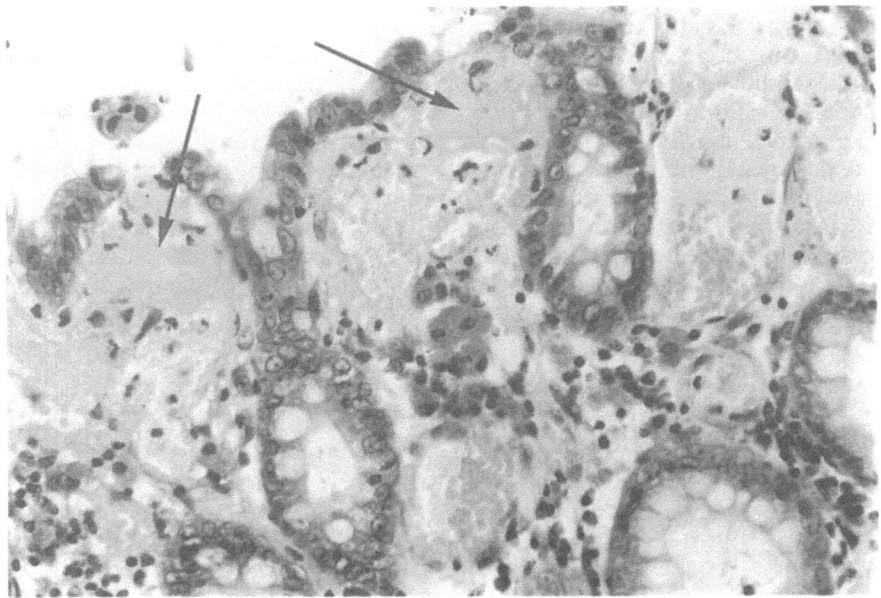

Fig. 5.13. Mucosal capillaries in RBD containing fibrin thrombi (*arrows*). (H&E ×280)

tion with the findings of Fajardo and Stewart (1973), these observations suggest that all vascular endothelium is radiosensitive and that permanent endothelial injury is a fundamental lesion of radiation damage to blood vessels.

Medial necrosis of arterioles is a well-documented sequel of irradiation in many tissues and Fonkalsrud et al. (1977) observed necrosis and fibrosis in the media of femoral arteries in their study. In contrast to endothelial damage which occurs immediately after exposure, lesions of the media often become apparent only after several weeks. It is well established that the supply of nutrients to the media of arterioles takes place by diffusion from the vessel lumen. Whilst a similar process provides nutrition to the inner part of the media of large arteries, the outer part is nourished by a capillary plexus arising from the vasa vasorum in the adventitia of the artery (Crawford 1977). On the basis of this, the morphological changes in the media of arterioles and arteries may result from impaired nutrition as a consequence of primary radiation damage to the endothelium of the vessel itself, or that of the vasa vasorum, rather than the direct effects of irradiation on vascular smooth muscle.

Progression of Vascular Lesions and Latency of Bowel Injury

These ischaemic complications in human bowel become manifest only after a latent period of time (Perkins and Spjut 1962; DeCosse et al. 1969; Russell and Welsh 1979; Localio et al. 1979; Berthrong and Fajardo 1981; Schofield et al. 1983). From studies in experimental animals, it seems that vascular injury occurs soon after irradiation and that the changes reach their maximum at 20–60 days (Eddy and Casarett 1968; Bosniak et al. 1969; Fajardo and Stewart 1973; Fonkalsrud et al. 1977). It is poorly understood why infarction or stricture formation does not occur at this time but it must be presumed that the damaged microvasculature is still able to meet tissue oxygen requirements and metabolic demands at this stage. The findings from several studies of human RBD indicate that the vascular lesions are active months or years after therapeutic irradiation (Sheehan 1944; Perkins and Spjut 1962; DeCosse et al. 1969; Localio et al. 1979; Berthrong and Fajardo 1981). Using vascular morphometry it has been shown that the degree of medial hypertrophy and intimal thickening is directly related to the time interval between the administration of radiotherapy and the onset of bowel symptoms (Carr et al. 1985a) (Table 5.2). On the basis of these observations it must be postulated that increasing vascular obliteration occurs due to the progression of vascular changes which ultimately compromises the microcirculation to a critical level at which ischaemia becomes inevitable.

Experimental Studies of the Microvasculature and Pathogenesis of Radiation Bowel Disease

Intravascular Studies in Experimental Animals

Histological examination gives a less clear view of the vascularisation of the bowel than intravascular studies using radiographic contrast medium. Microradiography of excised specimens gives excellent visualisation of the intramural vasculature and whilst it has been used in animals, the method has been little employed to study RBD in man. This technique was originally used by Eddy and Casarett (1968) to study the effects of small vessel disease on overall tissue vascularity in irradiated segments of rat small intestine. They demonstrated vessel occlusions and a patchy reduction in vascularity of the bowel wall which occurred within the first week after exposure. More recently, similar alterations in the microvasculature of the cat intestine were observed by Eriksson (1982) in the early post-irradiation period, but the subsequent appearances depended upon the initial dose of radiation administered. Whilst complete recovery followed low doses, high doses caused reduced vascularity and alterations in mucosal vascular pattern which persisted for 4 months. Bosniak et al. (1969) have examined the effects of different doses of irradiation on segments of canine bowel. They showed pronounced vasospasm at the time of exposure which was followed 4 to 7 weeks later by arterial occlusions and a decrease in the number of vessels in the irradiated segment. It seems that vascular injury occurs soon after exposure and that the severity and permanency of this are related to the initial dose of radiation.

Intravascular Studies in Human Radiation Bowel Disease

The later effects of radiation on the microvasculature in human bowel have received less attention although Denker et al. (1972) studied patients with bowel symptoms after pelvic radiotherapy using mesenteric angiography. They demonstrated reduced vascularity many months or years after therapeutic radiation. More detailed examination of the bowel microvasculature has been undertaken by the present authors (Carr et al. 1984b) in material from 19 patients who underwent resection of the terminal ileum and right colon, the recto-sigmoid colon or both these areas for RBD. Histologically normal areas of bowel from 45 patients who had resections for carcinoma of the colon and had not received radiotherapy were examined by the same techniques.

Fresh post-operative specimens were perfused with a 50% (weight to volume) solution of barium sulphate (Micropaque), through an arterial cannula which had been introduced into one of the mesenteric arteries. The barium sulphate was infused manually using a 60 ml bladder syringe at a pressure of 60–180 mmHg. Perfusion was continued until contrast medium appeared in the efferent mesenteric veins at which point the infusion was considered complete. The arterial cannula was removed and the cut edges of the bowel and mesentery oversewn to prevent leakage of contrast. After fixation of the specimens in 10% formalin for 48 hours, multiple transverse tissue blocks of the bowel wall were taken. These were obtained from each specimen at measured intervals throughout its length so as to obtain at least five blocks from each specimen. After routine processing, 5 μm sections were cut from each block and stained with haematoxylin and eosin (H&E) and Elastic van Geison (EVG). These sections were studied histopathologically so that the appearances could be compared with the microradiographic features from the same block. A 400 μm section was cut from the remainder of each block. These sections were sellotaped to a piece of thin card which was of the same dimensions as an industrex MX (Kodak) x-ray film. Using a cabinet x-ray system (Faxitron) a radiograph of the section was taken at 10 Kvp with an

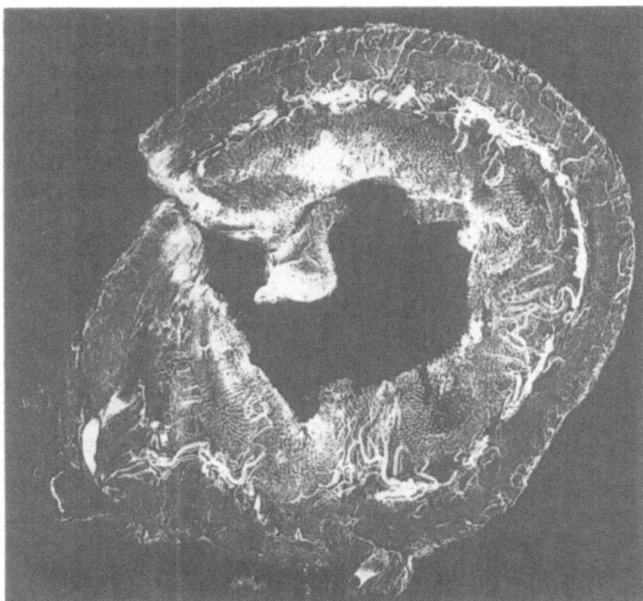

Fig. 5.14.   Microradiograph of normal terminal ileum. Shows dense vascular layers in submucosa and mucosa. (TS ×4)

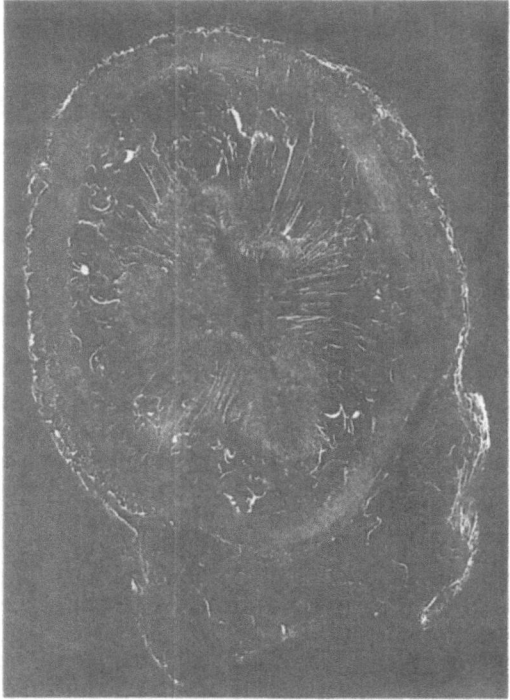

Fig. 5.15.   Microradiograph of radiation-induced stricture of the terminal ileum. Shows reduced vascularity of all the bowel wall layers. (TS ×4)

exposure time of 7.5 minutes. After development, the microradiographs obtained were studied under appropriate magnification using a microfiche projector and standard microscope.

Microradiographic Appearances

In normal small and large bowel, vascular density was most pronounced in the mucosal and submucosal regions (Fig. 5.14). The large tortuous vessels in the submucosa gave rise to the smaller vessels which supplied the mucosa and muscle layer. The vessels in the muscularis propria formed a loose network of freely anastomosing vessels. In the colon, the mucosal capillaries were closely packed together and regularly arranged. In the ileum the vascular pattern of the villi was observed. This comprised a central arteriole which branched at the tip of the villus into a number of descending capillaries which formed a richly anastomosing vascular network on the surface of the villus. Vessels appeared completely filled and uniform perfusion with contrast medium was always observed in all layers of the bowel wall. Variations in luminal diameter of vessels were infrequent.

Alterations in microvascular architecture were present in all sections from radiation damaged bowel, but the appearances varied with the type of lesion. At the site of fully developed strictures a reduction in vascularity which affected all layers of the intestinal wall was present (Fig. 5.15). Individual vessels exhibited luminal irregularities, variations in diameter and terminated abruptly. Non-uniform perfusion of the section with contrast medium was observed. Histologically, these areas showed pronounced fibrosis in the submucosa and muscularis propria together with severe vascular changes. These took the form of occlusive fibrin thrombi in capillaries, together with severe and sometimes occlusive intimal fibrosis in the small intramural arteries and veins.

In sections taken from sites adjacent to perforation and fistulae, sharply demarcated areas of the bowel wall which contained no contrast medium were present (Fig. 5.16). These avascular zones were either localised to part of the bowel wall or were transmural in distribution. When extensive, almost the entire circumference of a segment of intestinal wall was affected (Fig. 5.17). Focal or transmural infarction in combination with fibrinoid necrosis and thrombosis of vessels were found in these areas on histological examination.

In sections taken from areas remote from the main lesion, there was straightening of the submucosal vessels and reduced vascularity was most apparent in the submucosa. These changes were associated with submucosal oedema and fibrosis and non-occlusive intimal fibrosis in small arterial vessels in the bowel wall.

The mucosal vascular pattern was abnormal and the severity of change paralleled the reduction in vascularity in the remainder of the section. In the colon, localised areas of capillary ectasia situated adjacent to normal areas of mucosa were a common finding (Fig. 5.18). In other areas, the mucosa showed a loss of the normal regular capillary arrangement where mucosal regeneration had occurred. The first obvious change in the small bowel mucosa was villous blunting and was seen in sections distant from the stricture or perforation. In more severely affected sections, abnormal villi were seen showing ectatic vessels and a reduction in the villous capillary network (Fig. 5.19). In both the small and large bowel, there were areas of mucosa which were not perfused with contrast

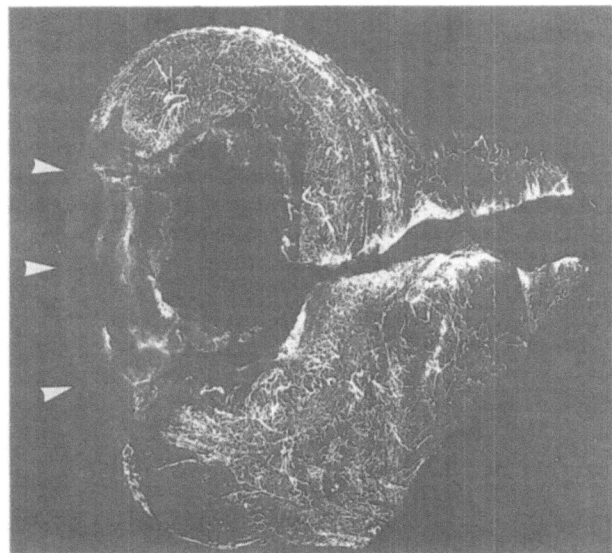

Fig. 5.16

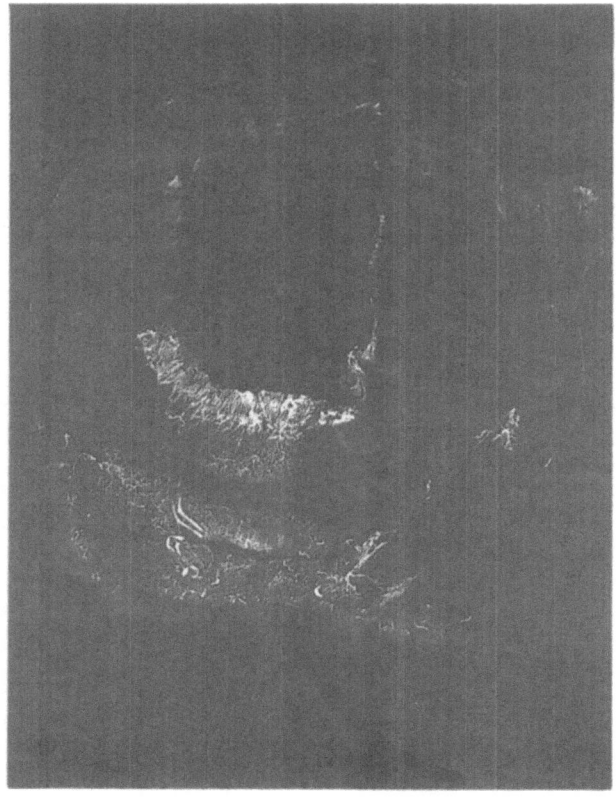

Fig. 5.17

Fig. 5.16. Microradiograph of radionecrosis of terminal ileum. Shows transmural avascular zone (*arrow heads*). (TS ×4)

Fig. 5.17. Microradiograph of radionecrosis of terminal ileum. Extensive avascularity of the bowel wall. (TS ×4)

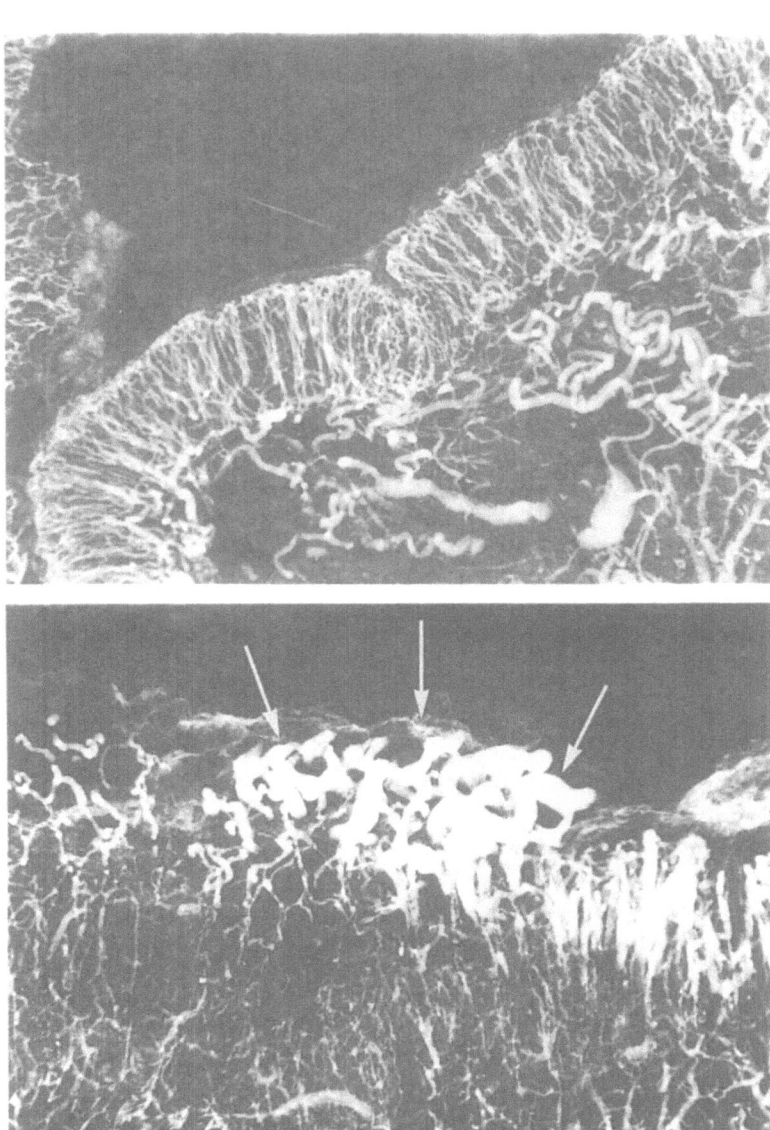

Fig. 5.18. Microradiographs comparing normal colonic mucosa (*top*) with that in RBD (*bottom*). The latter shows telangiectasia (*arrows*) of mucosal capillaries. (TS ×50)

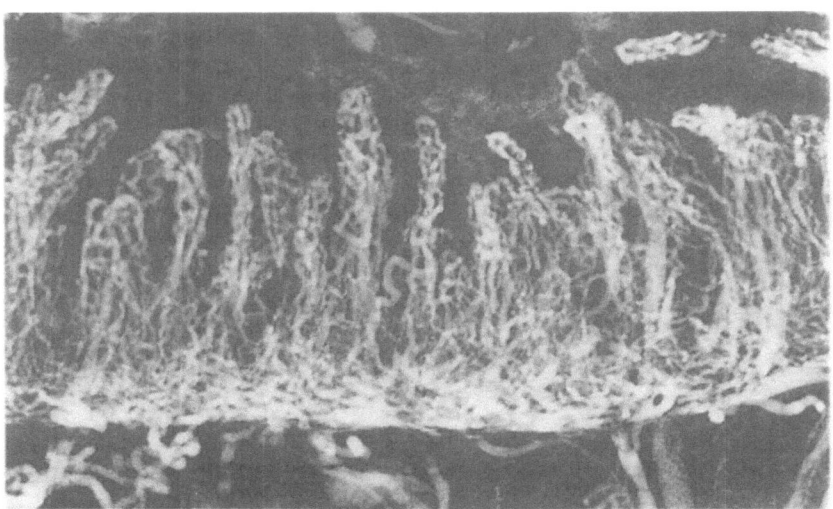

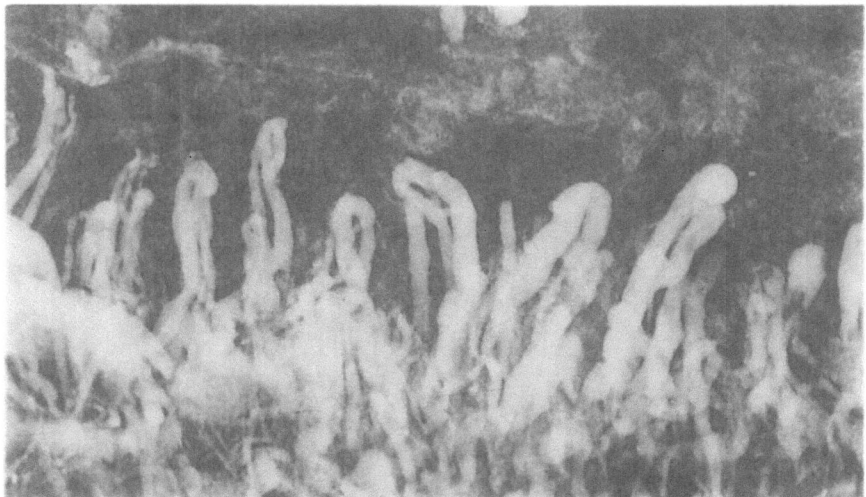

Fig. 5.19. Microradiographs of normal terminal ileum mucosa (*top*) and that in RBD (*bottom*). The villi in RBD show ectatic capillaries with a reduction in the surface capillary network. (TS ×80)

medium (Fig. 5.20). Capillary microthrombi were present in these mucosal vessels with or without accompanying mucosal necrosis.

Quantitative Assessment of the Microvasculature (Fluorescent X-ray Analysis)

Small samples of tissue (2×2 cm) were obtained from areas immediately adjacent to the points at which the blocks for histopathological and microradiographic

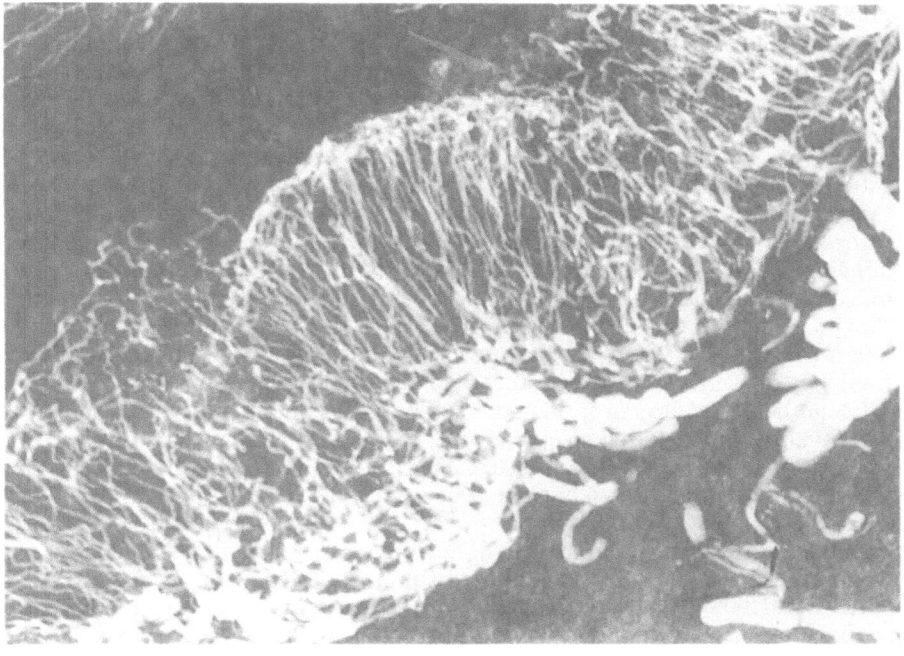

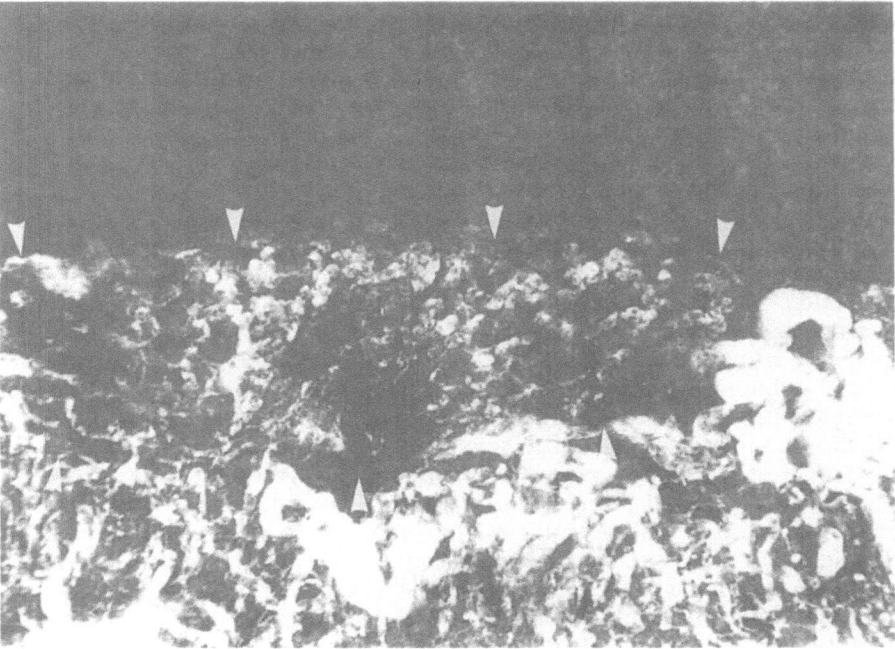

Fig. 5.20.   Microradiograph of normal colonic mucosa (*top*) compared with that in RBD (*bottom*) which shows an area of mucosa which has failed to perfuse with contrast medium (*arrowheads*). (TS ×80)

examination were taken. At least five samples from each specimen were studied. Each sample was dissected into a preparation consisting of mucosa-submucosa and a preparation comprising muscularis propria in order to estimate barium concentration and hence fractional microvascular volume in the whole sample and each bowel wall layer by fluorescent x-ray analysis (Carr et al. 1984c). Each sample of whole bowel, muscularis propria and mucosa-submucosa was exposed to 140 keV rays. The induced barium fluorescence was measured at 47 keV. The 90° scatter from the sample at 140 keV, which is a measure of tissue volume, was also recorded. The ratio of the number of counts obtained at 47 keV to those obtained at 140 keV for any given sample of whole bowel wall, muscularis propria or mucosa-submucosa was used as a measure of barium concentration (Carr et al. 1985c).

The mean value obtained for barium concentration in whole tissue samples of normal bowel wall was 2.031 ± 0.546%. Barium concentration was 1.315 ± 0.467% in the muscularis propria and 2.565 ± 0.726% in the mucosa-submucosa. The ratio between barium concentration in the mucosa-submucosa to that in the muscularis propria was 2.083 ± 0.654. The radiation group showed a highly significant reduction in mean barium concentration of the whole samples (1.004 ± 0.217%), the muscularis propria (0.677 ± 0.181%) and the mucosa-submucosa (1.209 ± 0.285%) when compared with the control group. The value for the ratio of barium concentration in the mucosa-submucosa to that in the muscularis propria was 1.905 ± 0.573, which did not differ significantly from that in the control group. The findings from this study confirm the subjective impression of reduced vascularity at the site of RBD and lend support to the hypothesis that the occlusive lesions of the small intramural vessels found in human RBD produce a profound reduction in microvascular space and ischaemia.

The sites of most severe injury after pelvic radiotherapy for carcinoma of the cervix, in which an intracavitary radiation source is employed, are the upper rectum and distal sigmoid colon (Perkins and Spjut 1962; DeCosse et al. 1969; Kott et al. 1971; Palmer and Bush 1976; Localio et al. 1979; Schofield et al. 1983). Overt injury to the small intestine is less common, but when it does occur it is usually situated 6–10 cm from the ileocaecal valve (Kott et al. 1971; Marston 1977; Carr et al. 1984b). It seems probable that injury at these sites is caused by the intracavitary radiation source. Lesions may occur in the mid and lower rectum and Todd (1938) in his monograph stressed that slipping of the intrauterine or intravaginal applicators is an important factor in the production of this type of injury. By contrast, Russell and Welsh (1979) found that damage occurring after external radiotherapy alone, used in the treatment of carcinoma of the bladder, was frequently situated higher in the sigmoid colon. In all these locations severe reductions in microvascular space have been demonstrated.

DeCosse et al. (1969) have stressed that the degree of involvement from radiation damage is far more extensive than is apparent on gross inspection. In order to investigate this hypothesis the relationship between the site of the specimen from which individual tissue samples were taken and barium concentration has been examined (Carr et al. 1984c; Carr 1985).

Six right hemicolectomy specimens, which had been removed for necrosis or perforation of the terminal ileum, were examined. All six patients had originally received combined intracavitary and external radiotherapy. Five normal specimens of terminal ileum and caecum were studied for comparison. Tissue samples were obtained from each specimen at measured distances from the ileocaecal valve. There were no significant changes in sample barium concentration at different points along the normal terminal ileum and caecum. By contrast, tissue samples from RBD specimens showed a maximum reduction in barium concentration within 15 cm of the ileocaecal valve. Sample barium concentration remained below the 95% confidence limits of the control range from up to 50 cm proximal to the ileocaecal valve (Fig. 5.21a,b).

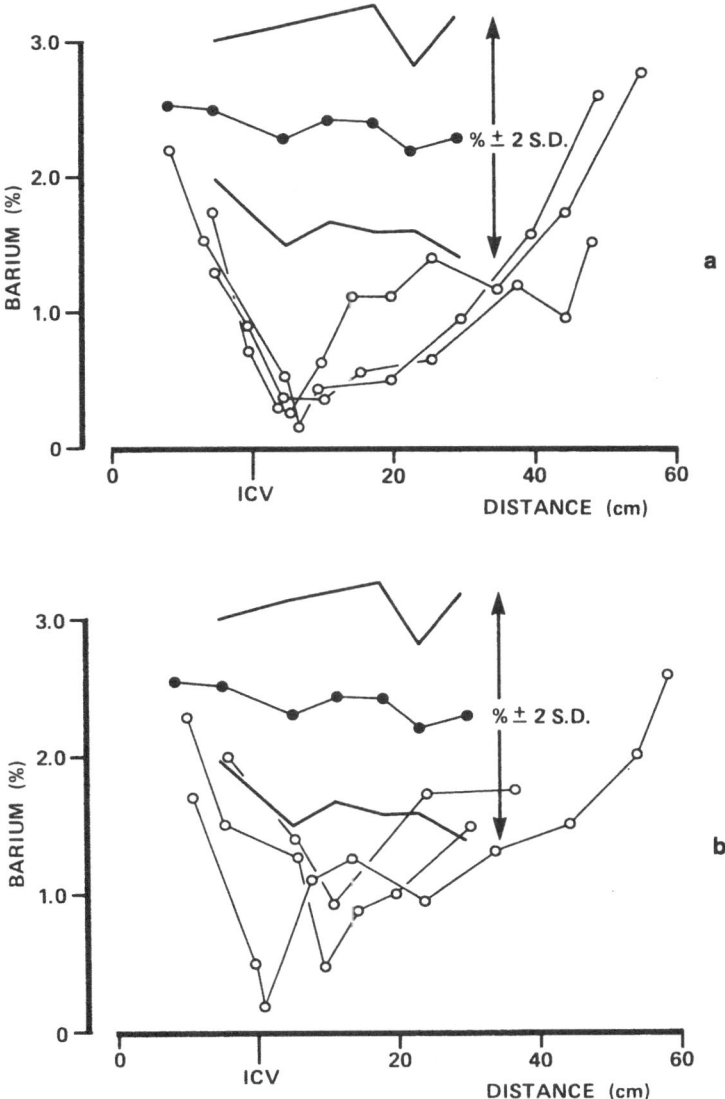

Fig. 5.21.a,b The relationship between linear distance (cm) and sample barium concentration (%) in normal terminal ileum (*solid circles*) and in RBD (*open circles*). *ICV* = ileocaecal valve.

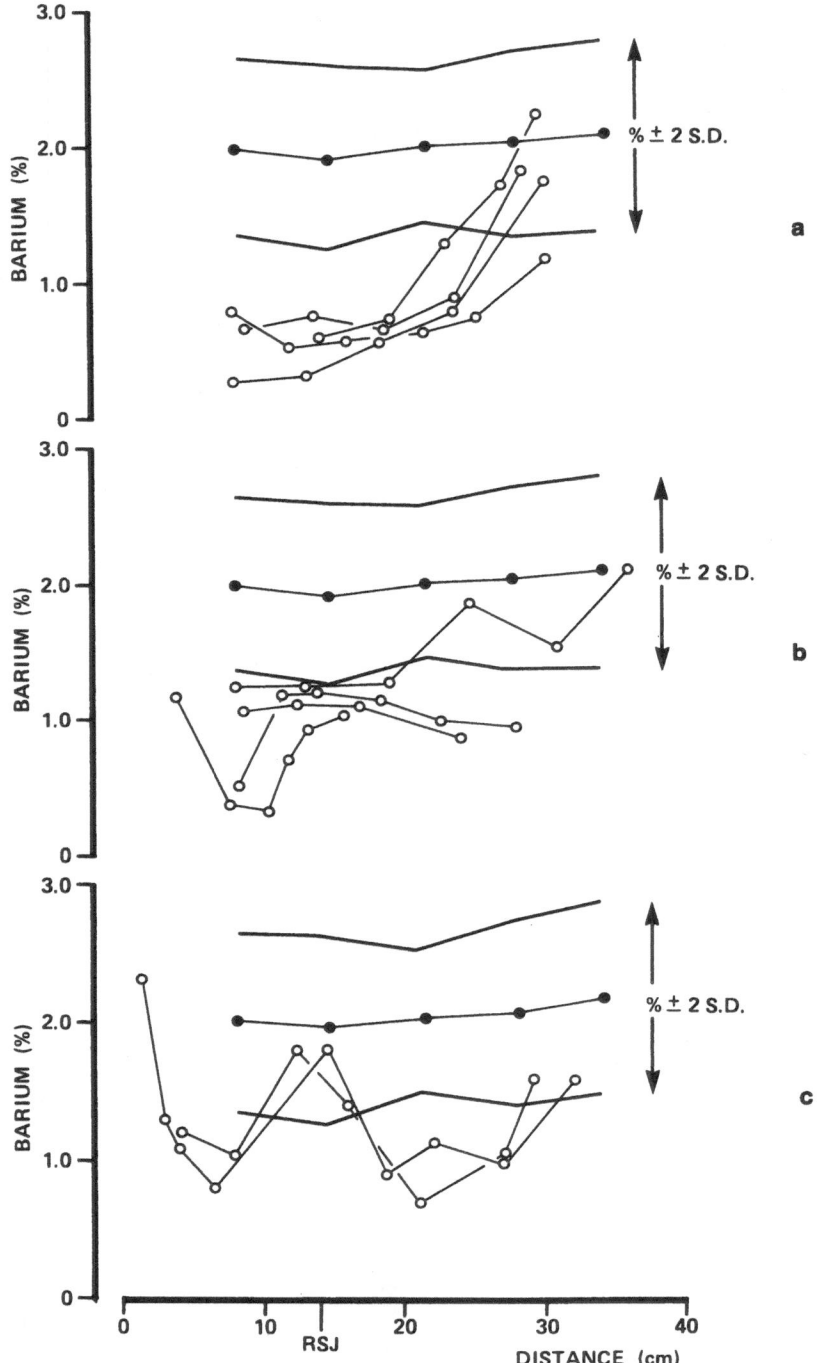

Fig. 5.22

Fig. 5.22.a,b,c Relationship between linear distance (cm) and sample barium concentration (%) in normal colon (*solid circles*) and in RBD of the rectosigmoid colon (*open circles*) produced by combined intracavitary and external radiotherapy. *RSJ* = rectosigmoid junction.

◄───

Fourteen specimens of radiation-damaged rectosigmoid colon and five control specimens were examined in a similar way, using the anorectal junction or rectosigmoid junction as a reference point. There was no significant change in tissue sample barium concentration at different points in the normal rectum and sigmoid colon. In RBD, the relationship between barium concentration and the site from which samples were taken was dependent upon the type of radiotherapy which had originally been administered. Ten out of 14 patients had received combined intracavitary and external radiotherapy. Stricture or necrosis was present in 6 out of 10 of these specimens (Fig. 5.22a,b) and the maximum decrease in barium concentration occurred in tissue samples taken 10 to 14 cm from the anorectal junction at the site of the main lesion. Sample barium concentration remained below two standard deviations of the control group in the proximal sigmoid colon (Fig. 5.22a,b).

In the remaining two specimens from patients who received combined radiotherapy, a rectal ulcer was present in one and a recto-vaginal fistula in the other. The greatest reduction in sample barium concentration from these specimens occurred in the mid and lower rectum. The values then rapidly returned to within the normal range and declined again in samples from the sigmoid colon (Fig. 5.22c) producing two quite separate areas of reduced microvascular volume.

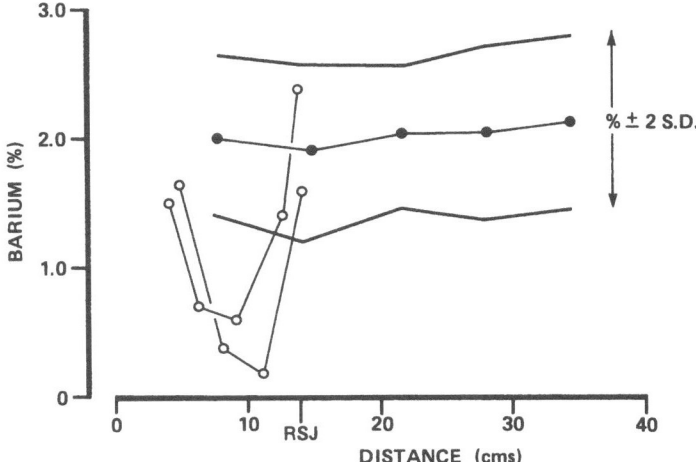

Fig. 5.23. Relationship between linear distance and sample barium concentration in normal colon (*solid circles*) and RBD of the rectosigmoid colon (*open circles*) produced by intracavitary treatment alone.

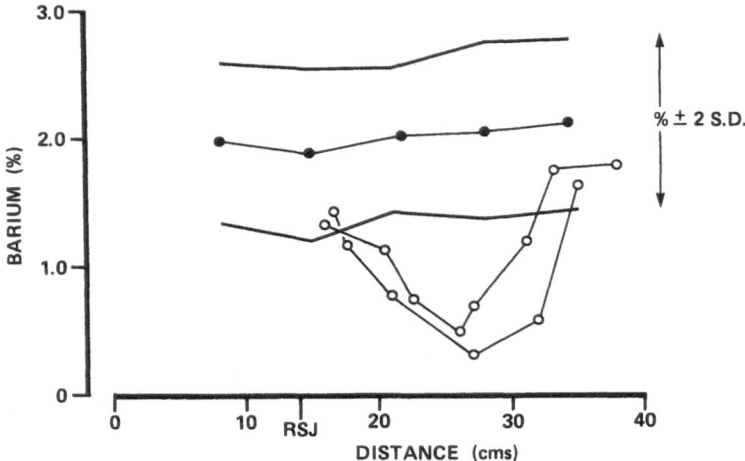

Fig. 5.24. Relationship between linear distance and sample barium concentration in normal colon (*solid circles*) and RBD of the sigmoid colon (*open circles*) produced by external radiotherapy alone.

Two patients had received intracavitary treatment only and external radiotherapy alone had been administered in the remaining two patients. Barium concentration in tissue samples from these specimens exhibited a localised reduction. In specimens from patients who had been subjected to intracavitary treatment only this reduction occurred in the rectosigmoid region (Fig. 5.23) whilst in the external radiotherapy alone group, the reduction occurred in the sigmoid colon (Fig. 5.24).

It seems that in patients who received combined intracavitary and external radiotherapy, reduced vascularity is present at sites distant from the main lesions, in segments of small or large bowel which do not appear grossly abnormal. These findings have important surgical implications in that extensive resection may be necessary in order to remove all the affected bowel and thereby prevent anastomotic failure or progression of the disease. In addition, microvascular injury is confined to much shorter segments of bowel in patients who received either intracavitary treatment only or external radiotherapy alone. These findings support those of Johnsson (1976) who observed that RBD is more localised if it occurs after intracavitary irradiation alone, and indicate that more localised resection is adequate treatment.

References

Ashbaugh DG, Owens JC (1963) Intestinal complications following irradiation for gynaecological cancer. Arch Surg 87:100–105

Berthrong M, Fajardo LF (1981) Radiation injury in surgical pathology. Am J Surg Pathol 5:153–178

Bogomoletz WV (1976) Fibrin thrombi, a cause of Clindamycin associated colitis? Gut 17:483–487

Bosniak MA, Hardy MA, Quint J, Ghossein NA (1969) Demonstration of the effect of irradiation on canine bowel using in vivo photographic magnification angiography. Radiology 93:1361–1368

Carr ND (1985) The intestinal vasculature in health and in certain non-malignant diseases of the bowel. MD Thesis, University of Bristol

Carr ND, Schofield PF (1984a) The colonic microcirculation. In: Givel J-Cl, Saegesser F (eds) Colo-proctology. Springer, Berlin Heidelberg New York, pp 11–25

Carr ND, Pullan BR, Hasleton PS, Schofield PF (1984b) Microvascular studies in human radiation bowel disease. Gut 25:448–454

Carr ND, Schofield PF, Pullan BR (1984c) A method for the determination of microvascular volume in tissue samples Clin Phys Physiol Meas 5:21–27

Carr ND, Schofield PF, Hasleton PS (1985a) Vascular changes in radiation bowel disease. Histopathology 9:517–534

Carr ND, Holden D, Hasleton PS, Schofield PF (1985b) Platelet count in radiation bowel disease: an aid to diagnosis. Br J Surg 72:287–288

Crawford T (1977) Blood and lymphatic vessels. In: Anderson WAD, Kissane JMC (eds) Pathology 7th edn. CV Mosby Co., St Louis, p 880

DeCosse JJ, Rhodes RS, Wentz WB, Reagan JW, Dworken HJ, Holden WD (1969) The natural history and management of radiation induced injury of the gastrointestinal tract. Ann Surg 170:369–384

Denker H, Holmdahl KH, Lunderquist A, et al. (1972) Mesenteric angiography in patients with radiation injury of the bowel after pelvis radiation. Am J Roentgenol 114:476–481

Eddy HA, Casarett HGW (1968) Intestinal vascular changes in the acute radiation syndrome In: Sullivan M (ed) Gastro-intestinal radiation injury. Excerpta Medica Foundation, New York, pp 385–395

Eriksson B (1982) Microangiographic pattern in the small intestine of the cat after irradiation. Scand J Gastroenterol 7:887–895

Fajardo LF, Berthrong M (1978) Radiation injury in surgical pathology. Am J Surg Pathol 2:159–199

Fajardo LF, Stewart JR (1973) Pathogenesis of radiation induced myocardial fibrosis. Lab Invest 29:244–257

Fonkalsrud EW, Sanchez M, Zerubavel R, Mahoney A (1977) Serial changes in arterial structure following radiation therapy. Surg Gynecol Obstet 145:395–400

Johnsson JE (1976) Bladder and intestinal injuries following radiation therapy of carcinoma of the uterine cervix. Acta Radiol Ther Phys Biol 15:541–545

Kott I, Luça I, Kesla H (1971) Gastrointestinal complications after therapeutic irradiation. Dis Colon Rectum. 14:200–205

Localio SA, Pachter HL, Gauge TH (1979) The radiation injured bowel. Surg Ann 11:181–205

Margaretten W, McKay DG (1971) Thrombotic ulcerations of the gastrointestinal tract. Arch Intern Med 127:250–253

Marston A (1977) Focal ischaemia of the small intestine. Edward Arnold, London p 136

McGovern VJ, Goulston SJM (1965) Ischaemic enterocolitis. Gut 6:213–220

Ming Si-C, Levitan R (1960) Acute haemorrhagic necrosis of the gastrointestinal tract. N Engl J Med 2:59–65

Palmer JA, Bush RS (1976) Radiation injuries to the bowel associated with the treatment of carcinoma of the cervix. Surgery 80:458–464

Perkins DE, Spjut HJ (1962) Intestinal stenosis following radiation therapy. Am J Roentgenol 88:953–966

Russell JC, Welsh JP (1979) Operative management of radiation injuries of the intestinal tract. Am J Surg 137:433–442

Schofield PF, Holden D, Carr ND (1983) Bowel disease after radiotherapy. J R Soc Med 76:463–466

Sheehan JD (1944) Foam cell plaques in intima of irradiated small arteries (100 to 500 microns in external diameter). Arch Pathol 37:297–308

Todd TF (1938) Rectal ulceration following irradiation treatment for carcinoma of the cervix uteri. Surg Gynecol Obstet 67:617–631

Whitehead R (1971) Ischaemic enterocolitis. An expression of the intravascular coagulation syndrome. Gut 12:912–917

6. Treatment of Radiation Bowel Disease

P. F. Schofield

Prevention

Radiation bowel disease (RBD) predominantly arises from radiation therapy for pelvic malignancy and both the rectum and any bowel in the Pouch of Douglas or recto-vesical pouch are particularly at risk. The greater the biological effect of any treatment regime, the greater is the possibility of achieving cure of the tumour but also the greater is the potential for producing RBD.

Treatment regimes have to be carefully planned to maximise cure rates whilst minimising unwanted toxicity (see Chapter 1). Attempts to monitor the dose to the rectum by intrarectal recording do not appear to have been successful in reducing RBD (Bourne et al. 1983). It is prudent for the radiotherapist to recognise the risk factors for RBD such as hypertension, arterial disease, diabetes (DeCosse et al. 1969) and coincident chemotherapy (Danjoux and Catton 1979) and, to some degree, moderate the intensity of treatment in such patients. Of particular interest to the surgeon is the risk factor of previous pelvic surgery when a loop of ileum or sigmoid colon may be adherent in the pelvis and receive a high dose of radiation. For this reason, it seems wise when combined radiotherapy and surgical management are being used to construct schedules so that the radiotherapy is given pre-operatively. There is no doubt that post-operative radiotherapy carries much greater hazard (Zucali et al. 1987). It has been suggested that this hazard can be minimised at operation if the surgeon knows that pelvic radiotherapy is to be used subsequently by attempting to exclude bowel from the recto-vaginal pouch. Omentum has been used to produce a barrier but has not proved totally effective so that other methods are being explored. One of these has been to introduce a spacer made of dimethyl polyseloxane into the pelvic pouch at the operation. Durig et al. (1984) showed that this is feasible and without ill effects in a small number of patients but a further operation is necessary to remove the spacer. A different type of exclusion procedure, using a polyglycolic acid mesh across the inlet to the pelvis, has been shown to be effective in animal experiments (Devereux et al. 1984). This appears to be a possible method for use in clinical practice as the mesh is completely absorbable.

Treatment of Early Disease

Early changes, during or shortly after radiotherapy, are usually self-limiting but supportive measures are desirable. It has been suggested that the early acute reactions may be minimised by the use of prostaglandin E_2. The rectal instillation of a thiophosphate compound has been shown to have significant protective effect in animals (France et al. 1986). Patients with abdominal cramp and diarrhoea can usually be managed by dietary modification and drugs to affect intestinal motility. In children, who have had total abdominal radiotherapy for lymphoma or other malignancies, a low residue, low fat, no milk and gluten-free diet has been said to effect an "improvement" in symptoms (Donaldson et al. 1975). On rare occasions it is necessary to interrupt radiotherapy when the manifestations of acute proctitis or acute enteritis do not respond to medical management. A severe enteritis with abdominal pain and vomiting is a rare complication but can usually be managed by intensive non-operative treatment. This involves naso-gastric decompression, intravenous fluids and appropriate antibiotics.

The requirement for surgery at an early stage is extremely rare but may be necessary for an exacerbation of pre-existing bowel disease, particularly diverti-cular disease (Schofield et al. 1983). Severe diarrhoea and vomiting during radiotherapy is a cause for grave concern for, whilst it will usually settle by adequate medical management, surgery may become necessary because of an acute perforation or persistent septicaemia. This situation, although rare, carries a high mortality.

Treatment of Late Disease

Symptoms arising from late disease vary from very minor disability to major life-threatening disease. The categories of disease severity suggested by Pilepich et al. (1983) are shown in Table 6.1 and are useful in discussing the therapeutic options.

Table 6.1. Categories of disease severity suggested by Pilepich et al. (1983)

	Morbidity	Treatment
Grade I	Minor symptoms	None
Grade II	Symptoms not affecting lifestyle	Simple outpatient
Grade III	Symptoms affecting lifestyle	Blood transfusion Laser therapy Dilatations of strictures etc.

Grade IV	Severe symptoms	Major surgery:
		  proctectomy
		  cystectomy
		  colectomy etc.

Grade V	Fatal	

Medical Treatment

There appear to be no medical measures that materially affect the progression of late RBD. Sulphasalazine, steroids, anti-fibrinolytic drugs and dietary manipulation, both of a high residue and a low residue type are still used in the medical management of RBD but there is no objective evidence to support their use. Medical management, therefore, should be largely symptomatic and supportive. Such measures are justified because some radiation-induced problems are self-limiting. Gilinsky et al. (1983) showed that two-thirds of patients with minor rectal bleeding from rectal RBD settled within 18 months but that if the bleeding were more major or other symptoms occurred, surgery was frequently necessary. Symptomatic treatment with stool softeners, oral iron or blood transfusion for anaemia and appropriate analgesics for pain has a definite place.

On rare occasions, symptoms arise from bacterial overgrowth in the small bowel consequent upon stenosis. In severe strictures, surgery may be necessary to correct the abnormality but many of these patients can be managed medically (Beer et al. 1985). The specific treatments include cholestyramine for bile salt induced diarrhoea, antibiotics for bacterial colonisation and vitamin B12, by injection, when deficiency of this substance is demonstrated. In more general terms, nutritional support enterally can be used but patient tolerance of some elemental diets is poor. In planning dietary supplements, it is important to be aware that there is a high incidence of lactase deficiency in these individuals and that they tend to be intolerant of fat (Beer et al. 1985). For this reason, milk and milk products are unlikely to be well tolerated.

Preparation and Timing for Surgery

Parenteral nutrition in the more severe RBD may be a useful pre-operative preparation in those cases requiring elective surgery. Many patients present with a combination of sepsis and incomplete intestinal obstruction with definite evidence of systemic upset. Such patients rarely settle with conservative measures, and parenteral nutrition should be seen as a prelude to surgery. In patients with fistulae, pre-operative total parenteral nutrition is valuable but it should be noted that, in our experience, no radiation-induced fistula from bowel has closed on conservative management alone.

Since there are several distinct presentations of RBD, it is not easy to generalise about the indications for operation. Occasionally there is an absolute indication for emergency surgery because of total intestinal obstruction, free perforation or massive bleeding but this is unusual. In our practice, approximately 40% of patients present as semi-urgent cases with signs of sepsis, incomplete obstruction or a recto-vaginal fistula. The largest group present with abdominal pain and/or bleeding sufficient to cause significant anaemia. In this last group, some maturity of surgical judgement is required to determine the optimal timing of operative treatment. It is our experience that most of these patients will ultimately come to surgery and, unless a good response is seen from conservatism, the operation should not be delayed overlong. A recent review of the management of patients with fistulae lays down basic principles which can be used as guide lines for the management of all patients with severe RBD (Smith and

Table 6.2.   Treatment of severe RBD

Stabilise
Define extent of disease
Operation

DeCosse 1986). The management of patients is divided into three phases: stabilisation, definition of disease and definitive surgery (Table 6.2).

Stabilisation includes correction of fluid and electrolyte imbalance and anaemia and total parenteral nutrition. These may be life-saving and must take precedence over diagnostic procedures. The second stage is the definition of areas of bowel involved (see Chapters 3 and 4) and the third stage is the operative management.

Operative Management

It is surprising that at this time there is still not general agreement as to the best surgical technique to use in RBD (Table 6.3). Indeed, there is not even general agreement as to whether bypass or resection of an irradiated area is the best policy. It is suggested that bypass will rest the bowel and allow ulceration to heal (Anseline et al. 1981; Wobbes et al. 1984). Some recent papers have advocated bypass for ileal disease and shown this to be safer than resection in some hands (Lillemoe et al. 1983; Wobbes et al. 1984) but resection based on correct surgical principles carries little morbidity in ileal disease (Schofield et al. 1986). It should be noted that many believe that RBD is progressive even if the bowel is defunctioned (Rubin 1984). When a colostomy is made to defunction the involved rectum it is rare for the situation to improve sufficiently to allow the colostomy to be closed without resection (Anseline et al. 1981). Provided well-vascularised tissue can be obtained after resection there is no contraindication to excisional surgery with primary anastomosis (Gazet 1985; Schofield et al. 1986; Galland and Spencer 1987).

Table 6.3.   Operations for RBD

Site	Operation	
	Defunction	Resection
Ileum	(a) Exclusion bypass (b) Exclusion and anastomosis	Ileo-caecal resection
Sigmoid colon	Colostomy	Sigmoid resection + colo-rectal anastomosis
Rectum	Colostomy	(a) A-P resection of rectum (b) Proctectomy + colo-anal anastomosis

Ileal Disease

On rare occasions surgery is necessary for acute enteritis with perforation. Such patients with a free perforation should not have a primary anastomosis because the extent of the disease is difficult to define. A resection with exteriorisation of the segments is the safest procedure, leaving reconstruction to be carried out when the acute reaction and illness are overcome.

In late ileal RBD we have advocated that there should be a wide excision of the involved small bowel because of the diffuse nature of the radiation damage. We usually find it appropriate to resect 50–60 cm of small bowel so that we are well above obvious RBD and into well-vascularised small bowel (Carr et al. 1984). An extensive colonic resection is not necessary as the ascending colon has not been irradiated and hence has normal vasculature. If an adequate resection is carried out there seems to be little greater risk of leakage than from other small bowel anastomoses, the incidence of leakage varying from 0 to 6% in a recent series (Schofield et al. 1986). The terminal ileum may be involved alone but in a significant minority of cases there is also injury to the sigmoid colon or rectum. It is important to correct the recto-sigmoid lesions at the same time as the ileal lesion is resected because distal obstruction would be a factor which would increase the chances of anastomotic leakage. The fear of producing significant short bowel syndrome has been overexaggerated and although a few of our patients have some diarrhoea it has rarely proved to be a disabling symptom. We also have no patients who have required long-term parenteral nutrition. Division of adhesions, oversewing of perforative lesions and local resection are dangerous operations and should be avoided. It seems probable that the high anastomotic leakage rates reported from earlier series are due to carrying out an inadequate resection (Galland and Spencer 1986).

The indications for bypass are rare. Although mobilisation of the involved ileum is frequently difficult it is usually possible with experience and patience. Some have found that on rare occasions the small bowel is so adherent that mobilisation is felt to be unwise and an exclusion bypass has been used instead of resection but in our view this is a less satisfactory procedure as the defunctioned loop may produce problems in the early or later post-operative phases.

Colonic Disease

Colonic disease may present as a procto-sigmoiditis with bleeding or as a chronic perforation with abscess or as a fistula. Each of these clinical presentations requires rather different handling.

Rectal Bleeding. This is the commonest presentation of large bowel RBD but the one in which surgical treatment is least likely to be necessary. Often the patient can be managed by the simple measures of avoiding constipation and the use of stool softeners. In minor but persistent rectal bleeding, successful control has been achieved by endoscopic YAG laser therapy (Ahlquist et al. 1986).

Radical surgery becomes necessary for massive bleeding, persistent bleeding requiring repeated blood transfusion or bleeding associated with chronic perforative disease. Since the bleeding arises from the rectum or sigmoid colon in these cases, rectal excision is required. In the past, we have found that abdomino-perineal excision of the rectum has always controlled the bleeding but in recent years we have moved to restorative resection using a colo-anal anastomosis and this has proved equally effective (Schofield et al. 1986) (Fig. 6.1).

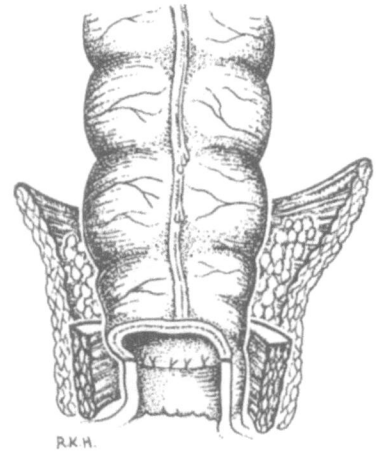

R.K.H.

Fig. 6.1. Colo-anal anastomosis: diagram with omission of anterior wall of anus to demonstrate posterior suture line. The sutures are inserted transanally.

Chronic Perforation with Abscess. Some of these patients present as urgent cases but it is usually possible to spend some time pre-operatively producing some stabilisation by correcting gross anaemia and fluid and electrolyte upset. Many patients have a profound nutritional deficiency with weight loss and a low serum albumin but it is rarely feasible to institute meaningful parenteral nutrition pre-operatively because it is desirable that surgery should be undertaken with reasonable haste to eliminate the sepsis. It will be apparent that individual patients present different problems and on a few occasions time spent in parenteral nutrition is justified.

The best operative management depends on the localisation of the RBD, the extent of the sepsis and the general condition of the patient. However, in all cases we believe that resection of the affected bowel is mandatory. The upper extent of the resection gives no great problem as the whole of the left colon can be mobilised, allowing the sigmoid loop and rectum to be completely removed. The difficulty lies in knowing where the distal line of resection should be. It is possible that the use of a laser doppler flow meter (Rotering et al. 1982) or an oxygen electrode (Sheridan et al. 1987) might help to define the vascularity in the distal rectum. In patients who have had combined intracavitary and external radiotherapy it is unsafe to leave any rectum and the resection should be taken down to the anal canal with an immediate colo-anal anastomosis and a protecting colostomy. When a single modality radiotherapy has been carried out, either intracavitary or external beam therapy, the lesion is often shorter and higher in the large bowel so that the lower rectum is spared and in these patients a low anterior resection is possible. The covering colostomy after colo-anal or low anterior resection is closed at about three months.

In a patient who is severely nutritionally depleted or in whom the sepsis is gross, consideration is given to closing the lower rectum and performing a Hartmann's procedure with the intention of a second stage colo-anal anastomosis. We would only do this under the most extreme circumstances as the second operation in these patients can be extraordinarily difficult so that in the majority of cases we carry out a primary colo-anal anastomosis.

Fistula. The ischaemic nature of late RBD may lead to necrosis of the bowel wall with fistulation. The common fistula is from the rectum to the vagina but fistulae may, on rare occasions, be from the sigmoid colon to the bladder or to another loop of bowel. Fistulae to the bladder or to other loops of bowel are not discussed further as they are managed by the same principles as such fistulae produced by other causes.

The typical recto-vaginal fistula caused by radiation produces management problems which are unique because of the poorly vascularised tissues in the region of the fistula. For this reason, simple closure is virtually never successful. There have been a number of operative strategies to overcome the difficulty. These include:

1. Permanent colostomy
2. Long-term colostomy with delayed repair of the fistula and subsequent colostomy closure.
3. Abdomino-perineal excision of the rectum.
4. Total rectal resection using colo-anal repair as a primary procedure with or without colostomy.

In considering these various options, the surgeon naturally wishes to avoid permanent colostomy. Simple colostomy has the advantage that it leaves the way open for subsequent repair of the fistula when it is "mature" and the patient is in a better state. It has the disadvantages that the necrotic inflammatory process tends to persist despite the defunctioning procedure and the patient has the disability of a colostomy for a year or more. However, the results reported from colostomy with delayed repair are interesting. Various methods of dealing with the fistula have been reported. The most successful appear to be the Martius technique of local repair, gracilis interposition and the utilisation of colon by an abdomino-vaginal repair. The Martius repair (Martius 1929) involves mobilisation of the bulbo-cavernosus fat pad from a labium major to act as a vascularised graft between the locally repaired rectum and vagina (Fig. 6.2). Some good short-term results have been reported. Boronow (1986) reported satisfactory results in 16 of 19 patients treated by the Martius method for radiation-induced fistula but gave no details of follow up. Aartsen and Sindram (1988) reported that although the Martius repair was satisfactory immediately, later breakdown occurred so that only 6 out of 14 patients so treated were without a colostomy at 10 years. It is possible that the gracilis muscle would provide a better vascularised interposition.

Bricker et al. (1986) adopt a different philosophy and attempt to repair the fistula by the use of mobilised colon after a period of defunction. They lay great emphasis on the fact that their method does not require full mobilisation of the rectum and have several different strategies for closing the fistula, depending on level. For the full details of their techniques it is necessary to read the original papers (Bricker and Johnston 1979; Bricker et al. 1981).

Our policy has been to resect the radiation damaged bowel, whatever the level of the fistula. Resection can be technically difficult but it is almost always possible for the skilled operator. Abdomino-perineal excision of the rectum undoubtedly cures the fistula but at the price of a permanent colostomy. We still consider this to be the procedure of choice if the sphincter mechanism is damaged.

In many instances, however, there is a better reconstructive alternative. For a very high fistula, a low anterior resection can be carried out but in the more usual fistula to the mid or low vagina restoration of intestinal continuity is by colo-anal

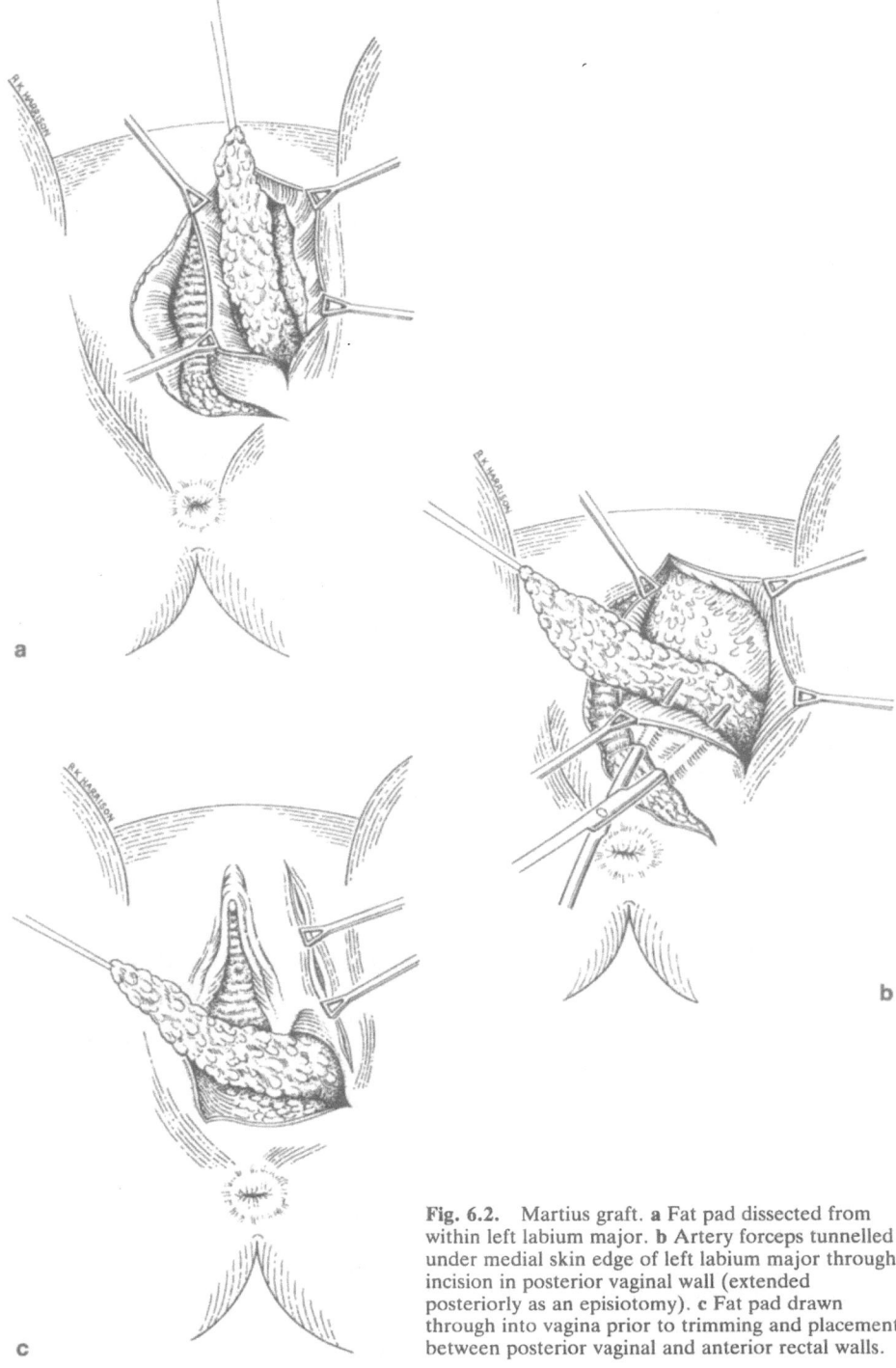

Fig. 6.2. Martius graft. **a** Fat pad dissected from within left labium major. **b** Artery forceps tunnelled under medial skin edge of left labium major through incision in posterior vaginal wall (extended posteriorly as an episiotomy). **c** Fat pad drawn through into vagina prior to trimming and placement between posterior vaginal and anterior rectal walls.

anastomosis. In this, the rectum and lower sigmoid colon are excised but the muscle of the lower rectum below the levator ani is preserved, stripping the rectal mucosa down to the dentate line. The dissection is usually remarkably bloodless. The rectal dissection must be especially meticulous so that it is freed from the vagina but the fistula itself is not closed. The descending colon is fully mobilised with high division of the inferior mesenteric artery, its upper left colic branch and the inferior mesenteric vein, together with full mobilisation of the splenic flexure. This allows the descending colon to be mobilised sufficiently to reach the anal verge. It has to be drawn through the levator ani. Sometimes the defect in the levator ani is too narrow for this to be done conveniently, in which case careful anterior dissection, splitting the muscle fibres, can be carried out so that the colon can be delivered without undue difficulty. The colon can be anastomosed to the anal canal transanally using a series of full thickness interrupted sutures. If the resection is down to the dentate line it is possible to carry out the anastomosis without an anal retractor in position as the anal canal can be exposed by temporary everting sutures into the buttocks. Colo-anal anastomosis of this type was first described by Parks et al. (1978) and a large series with very good results was reported by Cooke and Wellsted (1986). These workers leave a larger muscle tube than in the method just described.

This has been a procedure which we have always covered with a colostomy of a defunctioning type and at two to three months subsequently closed the colostomy. Recently Barker (1985) has suggested that the procedure can be carried out satisfactorily without a colostomy and has reported excellent results.

Peri-operative Care

The patient is catheterised after induction. All patients have metronidazole 1.5 g and cefuroxime 1.5 g at the beginning of the operation. A midline incision is used in all cases as it leaves both iliac fossae available for stomas as necessary. At the end of the operation, peritoneal lavage with tetracycline solution 1 g per litre is routine. Antibiotics may be continued for some days after the operation. High pressure suction drains are used for 48 hours if there has been extensive dissection but otherwise the abdomen and wound are not drained. Abdominal wounds are closed in layers or en masse with Prolene. The skin is then closed primarily.

Immediate Management after Surgery

The patient is managed by nasogastric tube for 48 hours. Intravenous fluids are given as indicated. If pre-operative parenteral nutrition was undertaken it is continued for at least 7 days after operation but most patients do not require this. The bladder catheter is removed at 5 days and skin sutures at 10 days.

Complications (Table 6.4)

Major wound infection is uncommon but minor infection which does not delay discharge has occurred in 12% of patients. The serious complications of resection

Table 6.4. Complications of surgery

EARLY = SEPSIS	LATE = "RECURRENCE"
Septicaemia	(a) Radiation recurrence
Wound infection	urinary tract
Anastomotic failure	other areas of bowel
	(b) Tumour recurrence

are poor anastomotic healing causing faecal fistula or peritonitis, late stricture at the anastomosis, subsequent RBD and coincident or subsequent radiation urinary tract disease. Provided well-vascularised bowel is used and the anastomosis is protected by a colostomy there is little reason to fear anastomotic leakage. It should not be different from similar operations performed for different pathology. Some years ago, we had cases of late-developing recto-vaginal fistulae after low anterior resection which I believe were due to making an anastomosis to an inadequately vascularised rectum. We have not seen this problem with colo-anal anastomosis. Some degree of stricture formation after colo-anal anastomosis or low anterior resection has been observed but it rarely seems to produce symptoms.

Outcome on Follow Up

There have been relatively few data on the long-term morbidity and survival after surgery for RBD. Recently there have been some papers which have looked at the longer term and our own experience extends back over many years in an institution with systematic follow up (Galland and Spencer 1986; Schofield et al. 1986; Harling and Balslev 1988). A major cause of morbidity and mortality in these patients is further radiation disease, most often affecting the urinary tract but occasionally involving a second area of bowel. DeCosse et al. (1969) reviewed 100 patients with RBD and found that 55 of them had urinary tract injury which in 16 was severe. It has been suggested that patients who suffer from RBD may have a better outlook, as far as their tumour is concerned (Perez et al. 1984). We suspect that this may be true and that the excess mortality from radiation-induced disease is balanced by a lower mortality from the primary tumour.

Some years ago, a review of the reported results of treatment indicated that 36% of patients treated by resection and anastomosis had anastomotic leakage (Swan et al. 1976). There is no doubt that this was due to inadequate resection and our own results with more radical excision and primary anastomosis indicate that leakage is rare (Carr et al. 1984). A recent review from Finland contrasts the longer-term results of colostomy with the results of resection. This study shows an excess of late re-operations in the patients who had colostomy and concludes that colostomy could not be regarded as the preferred operative method because it did not prevent progression of the disease and was associated with a higher late complication rate (Mäkelä et al. 1987).

My own experience began some 30 years ago when, as a trainee, I was able to see the results of the policy of colostomy to defunction the sigmoid colon and rectum and bypass for ileal disease. My subjective impression was that these patients did not do well. I followed a group of 18 patients who had had colostomy for rectal disease. At 5 years only 4 of them (22%) were alive. The majority had died due to continuing radiation problems rather than recurrent disease and this survival compared unfavourably with the patients who did not have radiation morbidity. It became clear to me that the disease was progressive even when bypassed and no longer carrying the faecal load and for this reason we have pursued a policy of radical excision in almost all cases of RBD treated in the last 15 years. Using this policy, we find that survival has been improved and in carcinoma of the cervix differs little from the expected survival for patients without RBD.

The long-term effect of RBD on morbidity and life-expectancy has recently been evaluated by Harling and Balslev (1988). They show that the 10-year survival rate in patients suffering RBD is 52%, as compared with 58% for the subjects who did not have this problem after radiation. There seems to be a significantly worse prognosis, however, for those patients who present with a recto-vaginal fistula. The evidence from our long-term results and that of others leads us to believe that adequate local resection is the treatment of choice in all sites.

References

Aartsen EJ, Sindram IS (1988) Repair of the radiation induced rectovaginal fistulas without or with interposition of the bulbocavernosus muscle (Martius procedure). Eur J Surg Oncol 14:171–177

Ahlquist DA, Gostout CJ, Viggiano TR, Pemberton JH (1986) Laser therapy for severe radiation induced rectal bleeding. Mayo Clin Proc 61:927–931

Anseline PF, Lavery IC, Fazio VW, Jagelman DG, Weakley FL (1981) Radiation injury of the rectum. Ann Surg 194:716–724

Barker EM (1985) Endo-anal anastomosis without proximal stoma – a safe procedure. Br J Surg 72:S132–S133

Beer WH, Fan A, Halsted CH (1985) Clinical and nutritional implications of radiation enteritis. Am J Clin Nutr 41:85–91

Boronow RC (1986) Repair of the radiation-induced vaginal fistula utilizing the Martius technique. World J Surg

Bourne RG, Kearsley JH, Grove WD, Roberts SJ (1983) The relationship between early and late gastrointestinal complications of radiation therapy for carcinoma of the cervix. Int J Radiat Oncol Biol Phys 9:1445–1450

Bricker EM, Johnston WD (1979) Repair of postirradiation recto-vaginal fistula and stricture. Surg Gynecol Obstet 148:499

Bricker EM, Johnston WD, Patwardham RV (1981) Repair of postirradiation damage to colorectum: a progress report. Ann Surg 193:555–564

Bricker EM, Kraybill WG, Lopez MJ (1986) Functional results of postirradiation rectal reconstruction. World J Surg 10:249–258

Carr ND, Pullen BR, Hasleton PS, Schofield PF (1984) Radiation bowel disease. Gut 25:448–454

Cooke SAR, Wellsted MD (1986) The radiation-damaged rectum: resection with coloanal anastomosis using the endoanal technique. World J Surg 10:220–227

Danjoux CE, Catton GE (1979) Delayed complications in colo-rectal carcinoma treated by combination radiotherapy and 5-fluorouracil – Eastern Cooperative Oncology Group (ECOG) Pilot Study. Int J Radiat Oncol Biol Phys 5:311–316

DeCosse JJ, Rhodes RS, Wentz WB, Reagan JW, Dworken HJ, Holden WD (1969) The natural history and management of radiation induced injury of the gastrointestinal tract. Ann Surg 170:369–384

Devereux DF, Kavanah MI, Feldman E et al. (1984) Small bowel exclusion from the pelvis by a polyglycolic acid mesh sling. J Surg Oncol 26:107–112

Donaldson SS, Jundt S, Ricour C et al. (1975) Radiation enteritis in children: a retrospective review. Clinico-pathological correlation and dietary management. Cancer 35:1167–1181

Durig M, Steenblock U, Heberer M, Harder I (1984) Prevention of radiation injuries to the small intestine. Surg Gynecol Obstet 159:162–163

France HG, Jirtle RL, Mansbach CM (1986) Intracolic WR2721 protection of the rat colon from acute radiation injury. Gastroenterology 91:644–650

Galland RB, Spencer J (1986) The surgical management of radiation enteritis. Surgery 99:133–138

Galland RB, Spencer J (1987) Natural history and surgical management of radiation enteritis. Br J Surg 74:742–747

Gazet J-C (1985) Parks colo-anal pull-through anastomosis for severe complicated radiation proctitis. Dis Colon Rectum 28:110–114

Gilinsky NH, Burns DG, Barbezat GO, Levin W, Myers HS, Marks IN (1983) The natural history of radiation induced proctosigmoiditis: An analysis of 88 patients. Q J Med 52:40–53

Harling H, Balslev I (1988) Long-term prognosis of patients with severe radiation enteritis. Am J Surg 155:517–519

Lillemoe KD, Brigham RA, Harmon JW, Feaster M, Saunders JR, d'Avis JA (1983) Surgical management of small bowel radiation enteritis. Arch Surg 188:905–907

Mäkelä J, Nevasaari K, Kairaluoma MI (1987) Surgical treatment of intestinal radiation injury. J Surg Oncol 36:93–97

Martius H (1929) Sphincter und Harnröhrenplastik aus dem M. bulbocavernosus. Chirurgie 17:49

Parks AG, Allen CLO, Frank JD, McPartlin JF (1978) A method of treating post-irradiation rectovaginal fistulas. Br J Surg 65:417–421

Perez CA, Breaux S, Bedwinek JM et al. (1984) Radiation therapy alone in the treatment of carcinoma of the uterine cervix. II. Analysis of complications. Cancer 54:235–246

Pilepich MV, Pajak T, George FW et al. (1983) Preliminary report on phase III RTOG studies of extended-field irradiation in carcinoma of the prostate. Am J Clin Oncol (CCT) 6:485

Rotering RH, Dixon JA, Holloway GA, McCloskey DW (1982) A comparison of the He–Ne laser and ultrasound Doppler systems in the determination of viability of ischemic canine intestine. Ann Surg 196:705–708

Rubin P (1984) Late effects of chemotherapy and radiation therapy: A new hypothesis. Int J Radiat Oncol Biol Phys 10:5–34

Schofield PF, Holden D, Carr ND (1983) Bowel disease after radiotherapy. J R Soc Med 76:463–466

Schofield PF, Carr ND, Holden D (1986) The pathogenesis and treatment of radiation bowel disease. J R Soc Med 79:30–32

Sheridan WG, Lowndes RH, Young HL (1987) Tissue oxygen tension as a predictor of colonic anastomotic healing. Dis Colon Rectum 30:867–871

Smith DH, DeCosse JJ (1986) Radiation damage to the small intestine. World J Surg 10:189–194

Swan RW, Fowler WC, Boronow RC (1976) Surgical management of radiation injury to the small intestine. Surg Gynecol Obstet 142:325–327

Wobbes T, Verschueren RCI, Lubbers E-JC, Janssen W, Paping RHL (1984) Surgical aspects of radiation enteritis of the small bowel. Dis Colon Rectum 27:89–92

Zucali R, Gardani G, Lattuada A (1987) Adjuvant irradiation after radical surgery of cancer of the rectum and rectosigmoid. Radiother Oncol 8:19–24

Part 3
Urinary Tract Disorders

7. Predisposing Factors, Clinical Features, Investigations: Radiation Urinary Tract Disease

E. W. Lupton

Radiation urinary tract disease has been reported after the treatment of tumours arising from bladder, prostate, ovary, vagina, vulva, testicle, lymph nodes and the gastrointestinal tract. Most reports have been concerned with problems after radiotherapy for carcinoma cervix and indeed much of our own experience has been with patients treated for cervical cancer. The potentially affected organs are the lower ureters, bladder, bladder neck and urethra.

Immediate Reactions (Early Disease)

Mild lower urinary tract reactions to pelvic radiotherapy occur less commonly than mild bowel reactions. Nevertheless, symptoms indicative of a degree of cysto-urethritis are encountered but scarcely necessitate any treatment. Such symptoms include urinary frequency, urgency, nocturia, dysuria and haematuria. These early changes are generally transient phenomena and rarely pose a continuing problem. Indeed, there is believed to be no direct relationship between the presence of early disease and later complications (Kline et al. 1972). The lower urinary tract is, in our experience, more tolerant of the immediate effects of radiation for carcinoma cervix than is the lower intestine. After radiotherapy for carcinoma bladder, however, there is a higher incidence of early reactions. A severe early response is more likely if the bladder is "sensitive" because of infection, inadequate drainage, extensive tumours or wide areas of post fulguration scarring (Friedman and Lewis 1958).

Late Disease

As with radiation bowel disease, later complications in the lower urinary tract may occur at periods ranging from a few months to many years after therapy. The main urinary tract complications are set out in Tables 7.1 and 7.2. Renal parenchymal thinning and scarring as well as functional deterioration may result from dilatation of the upper urinary tract, whatever the pathogenesis of the distension. Rarely, there may be fistula formation between the lower ureter and adjacent structures. Bladder changes vary from mild cystitis to gross compound fistula formation involving the bowel and urinary tract. Radiation disease of the urethra, including inflammation and stricture, is uncommon but most likely after treatment for carcinoma of prostate or the urethra itself.

Table 7.1. Complications of pelvic radiotherapy: upper urinary tract

Kidney	Ureter	
	Dilated	Fistula
Pyelonephritis	Obstructed	Uretero-colic
Poor/non-function	Refluxing	Uretero-uterine
Hydronephrosis		Uretero-vaginal

Table 7.2. Complications of pelvic radiotherapy: lower urinary tract

Bladder	Urethra
"Cystitis"	Urethritis
Contracture/fibrosis	Stricture
Fistula – vesico-vaginal	Fistula
vesico-colic	
recto-vesico-vaginal	
vesico-perineal	
Bladder neck stenosis	

It used to be believed that most of the significant urinary tract complications of pelvic radiotherapy were due to the effects of recurrent or residual tumour (Sackett 1935). More recent reports have demonstrated that disorders attributable to radiation-induced changes are commoner than previously suspected. The distinction between radiation disease and recurrent tumour may be difficult and even biopsy may not exclude tumour recurrence. On some occasions, the distinction is only made with certainty at autopsy.

The incidence of urinary tract radiation disease has been found to vary considerably between reported series over the years. The rate of occurrence of late radiation problems also differs with the organ treated. As techniques of x-ray treatment improved, the incidence of complications was observed to decline (Everett 1939; Everett et al. 1949). Nevertheless, the incidence of urinary tract disorders reported in more recent series of patients treated for carcinoma cervix has ranged from 2.7% to 11.7% (Cushing et al. 1968; Kline et al. 1972; Villasanta 1972; Ruponen 1977; Unal et al. 1981). Our own series of 62 patients presenting in a four year period with significant urological disorders comprises a small proportion of the total number of patients treated by radiotherapy for carcinoma cervix (approximately 4%).

Reports on problems after treatment of carcinoma bladder have been more sporadic. Not surprisingly, the number of bladder problems is greater than the number of upper tract complications (Friedman and Lewis 1958; Bloedorn et al. 1962; Miller et al. 1964; Caldwell et al. 1967; Ram 1970). In our experience, the requirement for major urological surgery in proven radiation disease after treatment of carcinoma bladder is uncommon. There is a reported incidence of significant urinary tract disease after radiotherapy for carcinoma prostate and gastrointestinal tumours (DeCosse et al. 1969; Ray et al. 1973; Mollenkamp et al. 1975; Sewell et al. 1975; Dean and Lytton 1978; Fowler et al. 1979; Schellhammer and El Mahdi 1983). A recent series demonstrated a 29% incidence of urinary tract complications after megavoltage radiotherapy for carcinoma prostate (Lindholt and Hansen 1986).

The time of onset of both upper and lower urinary tract complications after completion of treatment has been found to vary somewhat between series. Cushing et al. (1968) reported the mean time to development of major urological complications, ascribed to radiotherapy, as 12.3 months. Underwood et al. (1977) stated that most radiation-induced ureteric injuries become evident between 1 and 3 months after treatment. Muram et al. (1981), however, found that the time to development of ureteric injury varied from 3 months to 14 years after treatment with a median time of 18 months. The peak incidence of development of bladder injuries has been reported as 2 to 3 years (Kottmeier 1964). In the same series there were no serious radiation injuries discovered more than 4.5 years after treatment. Nevertheless, Villasanta (1972) is correct in suggesting that all patients are at risk from complications of radiotherapy for at least 5 years after treatment. Our own series has included several patients presenting more than 5 years after treatment and one patient at 19 years after therapy.

Another consistent observation has been the "lag" in the appearance of bladder, compared with bowel, injuries (Twombly et al. 1952; Kottmeier 1964; Villasanta 1972). This is supported by our own results in that the majority of patients with both bladder and bowel changes developed bowel symptoms before urinary problems. The reasons for the longer resistance of the urinary tract to the effects of radiation, in most patients, are not well understood. It seems that urinary tract disorders are less frequent after pelvic radiotherapy than bowel problems (Kottmeier 1964), a fact which is borne out by our own findings. However, DeCosse et al. (1969) described 55 cases of urinary tract injury in 100 patients with radiation enteritis, of whom 16 had severe disease of the urinary tract.

Predisposing Factors

Two of the most important factors are the total radiation dose to which the pelvic structures are subjected and the intensity of the administered radiation (Everett et al. 1949; Kottmeier and Gray 1961; Liegner et al. 1962; Villasanta 1972). The relevance of these features is discussed more fully in Chapter 1.

The individual response of each patient is important. Some subjects react more sensitively than others and tissue damage is more likely to occur (Ram 1970).

Pelvic visceral ischaemia, which increases the possibility of radiation damage, occurs with the arteriolar narrowing of hypertension, arteriosclerosis and diabetes and also with a decreased cardiac output (DeCosse et al. 1969). Bladder changes especially have been found to be more frequent in older patients (Miller et al. 1964).

The presence of sepsis within the pelvis or lower abdomen is a troublesome accompaniment of radiotherapy for pelvic tumours. Infection may be intrinsic within the urinary tract or extrinsic from pelvic inflammatory disease or inflammatory bowel disorders, such as diverticulitis. The lower ureters are especially at risk from a greater fibrotic reaction in the presence of active salpingitis (Graham and Abad 1967). Kottmeier (1964) has recommended that radiotherapy should not be given for carcinoma cervix when the patient has an offensive vaginal discharge. Even quiescent salpingitis may be exacerbated by the effects of x-ray treatment. Similarly, it is advisable to avoid potential infection during the treatment of carcinoma bladder and prostate. Unfavourable situations include inadequate bladder drainage and an indwelling urethral catheter.

The performance of prior or subsequent pelvic surgery is strongly suspected as a contributory factor to the development of complications. The combination is thought to be more hazardous to pelvic organs than radiotherapy or surgery alone. Possible aetiological factors are denervation and damage to the blood supply. The ischaemia resulting from irradiation and tissue dissection impairs healing and delays the resolution of inflammatory processes, both of which increase fibrosis. Hysterectomy, particularly radical hysterectomy, has been reported by several authors to put patients at greater risk of complications from x-ray therapy for carcinoma cervix (Strockbine et al. 1970; Kaplan 1977; Kjorstad et al. 1983). Nieminen and Pollanen (1970) found that 20.6% of patients treated by radiotherapy alone suffered complications compared with 39.9% treated by surgery and radiation. With bladder tumours, transurethral resections in the three weeks prior to the x-ray therapy have been implicated in producing higher complication rates. It has also been recognised that multiple transurethral resections, prior to x-ray therapy, increase the likelihood of subsequent radiation damage (Schellhammer et al. 1986). Similarly, patients having previous suprapubic prostatectomies for benign enlargement have tolerated poorly x-ray therapy for subsequent carcinoma prostate whereas a transurethral resection during or after radiotherapy has been well accepted (Mollenkamp et al. 1975).

Finally, the extent of treated tumours plays a part in determining the degree of tissue damage. Large advanced lesions tend to produce more complications after treatment (Kottmeier and Gray 1961; Hiilesmaa et al. 1981).

Clinical Features

Symptoms and Signs

It was formerly believed that almost all the significant complications from pelvic radiotherapy were vesico-vaginal fistulae and obstructed ureters (Sackett 1935). It is clear from more recent reports and our own observations that "cystitis" is the most common urological problem resulting from pelvic radiotherapy (DeCosse et al. 1969; Villasanta 1972). Local lower urinary tract symptoms predominate during the initial stages of late disease. Frequency of micturition may be mild, the patient perhaps voiding every 80–90 minutes. More severe frequency and urgency may produce an incessant desire to void with regular 15–20 minute attempts. The urge to void is often urethral but there may be suprapubic discomfort because of a reduction in functional bladder capacity as the result of vesical fibrosis. There may be associated nocturia. Dysuria can occur intermittently because of recurrent urinary infection or continuously because of significant bladder urothelial congestion, inflammation, necrosis and slough. There may be discolouration of the urine with the passage of blood and/or debris. A generalised pelvic pain may accompany urinary symptoms. It is common for women after treatment of carcinoma cervix to have vaginal discharge, bleeding (possibly post-coital) and dyspareunia.

Urinary incontinence may be present and both stress and urge incontinence have been encountered. Stress leakage after x-ray treatment occurs because of fixation of pelvic structures as well as shortening and fibrosis of the urethra which remains open even at rest. Muscles of the pelvic diaphragm are less effective after radiotherapy because of fibrosis and are less able to support the intrinsic urethral sphincter mechanism during rises of intra-abdominal pressure such as with coughing. Urge incontinence is an extension of urgency and frequency due to various degrees of cystitis or reduced bladder capacity. Continuous incontinence may be symptomatic of urinary fistula, for example, uretero-uterine, uretero-vaginal or vesico-vaginal.

Pneumaturia and persistent urinary infections suggest a vesico-rectal or vesico-colic fistula. Loin pain may indicate the presence of ureteric obstruction or perhaps pyelonephritic changes. Severe disease may result in weight loss, malaise, anorexia and the symptoms of septicaemia. By contrast, quite marked affectation of the lower or upper urinary tract can produce little symptomatic disturbance of the patient, for example, small capacity bladders with normal voiding patterns or symptom-free upper urinary tract dilatation.

The physical examination of the patient with radiation urinary tract disease may not be very revealing. General changes become apparent if there has been a significant amount of pelvic necrosis and infection. The patient may be wasted, asthenic and there is the suspicion of recurrent tumour. Anaemia, dehydration and pyrexia are sometimes present. Abdominal examination is seldom fruitful unless peritonitis is present or there are associated bowel problems such as intestinal obstruction. An enlarged kidney associated with ureteric obstruction may be palpable but this is rare.

Pelvic examination is often useful. In female patients the vagina is commonly shortened and stenosed especially following radiotherapy for carcinoma cervix. There may be other local vaginal problems such as bleeding, discharge and cervical ulceration and/or necrosis. The distinction from recurrent tumour may be difficult and biopsy is desirable. Pelvic thickening and rigidity of pelvic structures are often better felt by rectal rather than vaginal examination. The presence of a pelvic mass need not necessarily indicate recurrent tumour especially in patients with early pelvic complications of x-ray therapy. Urine leakage may be seen per vaginam or per rectum. The distinction must be made between urine leakage per urethram due to stress incontinence and the presence of a vesico-vaginal fistula. A fistula may be felt or suspected from induration around the vaginal wall defect even if urine leakage is not confidently identified.

Upper Urinary Tract Disorders

See Table 7.1. Pelvic radiotherapy can directly affect the integrity and structure of the lower ureters. Scarring, inelasticity and stricture formation may produce a genuine obstruction to urine flow. Vesico-ureteric reflux and, more rarely, a fistula from the lower ureter may develop. Whichever of these occurs, the proximal upper urinary tract may become dilated. The end-results of these processes are, potentially, renal parenchymal atrophy or scarring, loss of renal function and perhaps even a pyonephrosis to further compound the problem (Cushing et al. 1968).

Ureteric Obstruction

The incidence of ureteric injury after pelvic radiotherapy has changed with experience and refinement of treatment techniques. Everett (1939) found that 48% of 33 patients studied urologically after treatment of carcinoma cervix developed ureteric dilatation and in 15% "the obstruction" was severe. By 1960, Burns et al. had found considerable decline in the occurrence of ureteric stricture. They reported only one clinically significant stricture in a series of 295 patients. Since 1960, the incidence of ureteric dilatation attributable to radiotherapy for carcinoma cervix has been found to range from 0.26% to 4% (Kaplan 1977; Underwood et al. 1977; Shingleton et al. 1969). The reports of such injury following radiation to other pelvic organs are even more scanty. Although the clinical incidence of isolated ureteric injury is small in both symptomatic and sympton-free patients, it is well recognised that radiation-induced bilateral ureteric obstruction can lead to uraemia and death from renal failure (Altvater and Imholz 1960; Kirchoff 1960; Lupton and Barnard 1986, unpublished work presented at the British Association of Urological Surgeons, Autumn Meeting, Manchester, October 1986).

There is contention about the most frequent site of damage to the ureter. After radiotherapy for carcinoma cervix, it has been suggested that it occurs mostly at 4–6 cm above the ureteric orifice, where the ureter passes through the broad ligament (Kaplan 1977). This is the area where tumour invasion often occurs, where a high level of radiation is received and where parametritis with subsequent fibrosis is common (Villasanta 1972). Another finding has been a long, thread-like stenosis of the ureter from pelvic brim downwards (Altvater and Imholz 1960). A third alternative is a narrowing at the vesico-ureteric junction (Unal et al. 1981). In our experience, lower ureteric strictures may occur in any of these three sites but most of the strictures we have encountered were in the distal ureter within 5 cm of the ureteric orifice.

The distinction between ureteric dilatation due to radiotherapy and that due to recurrent or "residual" tumour is difficult. It has been suggested that most ureteric obstruction after treatment for carcinoma cervix is due to tumour extension and is an indication of a poor prognosis (Aldridge and Mason 1950; Burns et al. 1960). Muram et al. (1981), however, found that 12 of 34 patients (35%) with dilated ureters had radiation injury. If the dilatation was first noticed two or more years after treatment and was unilateral, it was more likely to be due to radiation damage than tumour. Furthermore, dilatation associated with treatment of early stage tumours was less likely to be due to persistent or recurrent malignancy than if there was an advanced tumour stage at presentation. It has been observed that ureteric injury due to radiation increases with tumour stage (Lang et al. 1973). Ureteric dilatation before or after radiotherapy need not necessarily herald a poor prognosis. Indeed, dilatation found at presentation may well improve after radiotherapy because of tumour shrinkage (Kottmeier 1964).

It has been postulated that the distinction between tumour-induced and radiation-induced lower ureteric strictures may be made on clinical grounds. Patients who complain of an associated proctitis or cystitis are more likely to have radiation disease. Those who present with pelvic pain or sciatica are more likely to have tumour recurrence (Zerbig et al. 1983).

Vesico-ureteric Reflux

Reflux may result from fixation of the intramural ureter and fibrosis round the ureteric orifice which becomes held in an open state. It may be more common than has so far been reported but has been described following radiotherapy for carcinoma cervix (Albrecht 1981) and in association with small capacity bladders after treatment of bladder tumours (Ram 1970). In our own experience, reflux is not as common a problem as stricture formation and does not often require treatment in its own right.

Ureteric Fistulae

Fistula formation can occur because of the close matting together of pelvic tissues after radiotherapy. Our own series of patients treated for carcinoma cervix has included cases of uretero-uterine and uretero-vaginal fistulae. However, the incidence of ureteric fistulae has been low in the experience of most authors. For example, Villasanta (1972) found only one case in 311 patients treated for stage III cervical carcinoma. Nieminen and Pollanen (1970) reported 13 such fistulae in a series of 640 patients treated for carcinoma cervix.

Lower Urinary Tract Disorders

See Table 7.2. The most common urinary tract complications of pelvic x-ray treatment involve the bladder (Ram 1970; Villasanta 1972). In their series of 500 consecutive cases treated for carcinoma cervix, Kottmeier and Gray (1961) reported a 20.8% incidence of bladder injury. The incidence of significant bladder complications after radiotherapy for carcinoma bladder has ranged from 5% to 15% (Miller et al. 1964; Schellhammer et al. 1986).

Cystitis

The effects of inflammation of the bladder range from mild frequency and dysuria to gross persistent urgency, frequency, haematuria and pelvic discomfort. Some patients may experience increasingly troublesome cystitis prior to the development of another problem, for example, a fistula. Despite the fact that some form of cystitis is the most commonly reported disorder, the incidence varies considerably between series. Hiilesmaa et al. (1981) and Chau et al. (1962) reported respectively 2% and 1.3% incidence of cystitis after treatment of carcinoma cervix. Ram (1970) described an 8% incidence of significant cystitis following radiotherapy for carcinoma bladder but Dean and Lytton (1978) found persistent cystitis in only 2 of 240 cases. The incidence of cystitis, albeit transient in some cases, has been reported as high as 41% after x-ray treatment of carcinoma prostate (Sewell et al. 1975). In the experience of most authors, however, the incidence of cystitis after treatment of carcinoma prostate is less than 5% (Schellhammer et al. 1986).

With severe inflammatory change, significant vesical haemorrhage may occur and can present a persistent and serious problem (Turner 1961). Indeed some haemorrhages have a fatal outcome (DeCosse et al. 1969). It is well recognised that bleeding occurs from extensive "telangiectasia" but it may arise from destruction of the mucous membrane (Riches and Windeyer 1960). Another factor is the possibility of unremitting bleeding from residual or recurrent tumour whose supplying blood vessels have been modified by the radiotherapy (Turner 1961).

Another manifestation of severe disease is the presence of bladder ulceration which has been well documented after treatment of carcinoma cervix and carcinoma bladder (Lenz et al. 1947; Bloedorn et al. 1962; Strockbine et al. 1970; Chau et al. 1962). Non-healing radionecrotic ulcers are believed to develop during the first two years after treatment. Haematuria associated with ulcers is sometimes profuse, persistent and dificult to control. The severity of radionecrosis is greater with infection and inadequate bladder drainage. Areas of slough may become calcified and eventually pieces may break away to form bladder stones. Recurrent bladder perforation has also been reported in association with chronic radiation cystitis (Golomb et al. 1986).

Bladder Contracture

This is a relatively common problem after pelvic x-ray therapy. Fibrous replacement of the vesical muscle may produce a low compliance, inelastic bladder wall. Patients may be symptom free but alternatively the inability of the wall to expand and accommodate normal volumes of urine may produce frequency, urgency, nocturia and suprapubic discomfort. Such contractures of the bladder may become significant some months after radiotherapy but may take several years to develop. A grossly contracted bladder with a small capacity may be associated with vesico-ureteric reflux when the ureters are narrow and indistensible in their pelvic course (Ram 1970).

Fistulae

Vesical fistulae indicate severe injury to the bladder and surrounding structures. The commonest fistula arises between bladder and vagina after treatment for carcinoma cervix. The incidence of vesico-vaginal fistula in this situation is between 1% and 2% (Cushing et al. 1968; Strockbine 1970; Villasanta 1972). Patients treated for early stage tumours are said to have little risk of developing a fistula (Kottmeier and Gray 1961). It is usual for patients developing a vesico-vaginal fistula to have had extensive central tumours or considerable vaginal involvement. Biopsy of a suspect but benign vaginal ulcer may precipitate a fistula (Boronow 1971).

A fistula may also form between bladder and rectum or bladder and colon. Rarely, an entero-vesical fistula may arise. A vesico-perineal fistula can occur after pelvic operations such as abdomino-perineal excision of the rectum. In the severely diseased pelvis, with much tissue destruction, necrosis and ischaemia, compound fistulae may develop. After abdomino-perineal excision of the rectum with hysterectomy a vesico-vagino-perineal fistula may develop. Even more troublesome are the combined bowel and urinary tract fistulae. Considerable management problems are encountered in patients with a recto-vesico-vaginal fistula or a vesico-vagino-colic fistula. Compound fistulae involving small and large bowel, bladder and vagina have been seen following treatment of carcinoma cervix in our series (see Appendix).

Bladder Neck and Urethral Problems

These disorders have mainly been recognised after radiotherapy for carcinoma prostate. Contracture of the bladder neck most often occurs if there has been previous prostatic or bladder neck resection (Mollenkamp et al. 1975). Other problems include prostatic calculi and fibrous fixation·of the distal urethral sphincter complex which may result in stress urinary incontinence. The urethra may become inflamed or strictured and, rarely, a urethral fistula may occur.

The incidence of urethral stricture after radiotherapy for carcinoma prostate ranges from 5% to 11% (Schellhammer et al. 1986). The chances of developing a urethral stricture increase if multiple pretreatment transurethral procedures have been performed (Ray and Bagshaw 1975).

Investigations

There are some investigations which are appropriate for all patients with radiation urinary tract disease. Other tests are more selectively requested. A list of potentially useful investigations is shown in Table 7.3 with two categories: (a) those which are commonly performed and (b) those less frequently required.

A midstream specimen of urine is routinely sent to check on the presence or absence of red and white cells as well as to detect any infection. A chest x-ray is performed mainly to exclude metastatic lung tumour and to aid the assessment for anaesthesia, if necessary. A haematological screen including erythrocyte sedimentation rate and platelets is useful. A change in platelet count associated with exacerbations of radiation bowel disease has been described in Chapter 4. Similar, although not so well-documented rises, have been seen during the acute phases of radiation disease of the urinary tract. Urea and electrolyte levels and creatinine clearance estimations are mandatory indicators of global renal function. A frequency-volume chart is a simple record kept by the patient of the

Table 7.3. Radiation urinary tract disease: investigations

(a) Routine	(b) Specialised
MSU	Ultrasound – upper urinary tracts/pelvis
Chest x-ray	CT scan – abdomen/pelvis
Full blood count	Micturating cystography
ESR	Video-urodynamics
Platelets	Antegrade pyelography
Urea and electrolytes	Pressure-flow studies
Creatinine clearance	Retrograde pyelography
Intravenous urogram	Fistulogram
Renogram (? diuresis)	Three swab test
Frequency/volume chart	
Cystoscopy/EUA	

number of voidings and the urine volume on each occasion. It provides an objective demonstration of frequency and the prevalence of leakage episodes.

One of the earliest radiological investigations is the intravenous pyelogram. As discussed in Chapter 3, much information is potentially yielded by this time-honoured study, especially with regard to the upper urinary tracts. Most ureteric injuries become evident during the first 3–5 years after radiation and regular follow-up urograms have, therefore, been recommended up to this time (Shingleton et al. 1969; Underwood et al. 1977).

Renography is a sensitive indicator of individual renal function and excretion. The radiation dose is very small which makes it particularly useful for serial appraisal. Diuresis renography helps determine the nature of upper urinary tract dilatation (O'Reilly et al. 1986).

Other potentially useful radiological investigations have been discussed in Chapter 3. Antegrade pyelography may be accompanied by pressure/flow studies to help determine the presence or absence of ureteric obstruction (Whitaker 1979; Lupton et al. 1985). Video-urodynamics may help evaluate urinary incontinence.

Cystoscopy is an almost mandatory investigation in patients with radiation urinary tract disease. Abnormal bladder findings range from the mildest mucosal inflammatory changes to gross and compound fistulae or negligible capacity bladders. The earliest feature of radiation cystitis is a typical pallor of the mucosa. Later changes include congestion, oedema and hyperaemia of the urothelium. The abnormalities may be confined to a certain area of the bladder or be generalised. A common feature is telangiectasia which is present to a degree in most bladders after pelvic radiotherapy. More severe changes include fibrosis of both muscle and mucosa as well as slough and ulceration from a severe ischaemic reaction. Haemorrhage may arise from congestion, telangiectasia and ulcerated areas. Still more severe mural damage causes the development of vesico-vaginal, recto-vesico-vaginal, vesico-colic, vesico-perineal and other fistulae.

It is often difficult to distinguish post-radiation changes in the bladder from recurrent tumour and, indeed, the former may significantly mask the latter. We have, on several occasions, received histology reports indicating the presence of tumour which was not obvious on cystoscopy. We would advocate biopsy of any suspicious areas and accept that on rare occasions a fistula may result from low posterior wall biopsy.

Accompanying the cystoscopy is an examination under anaesthesia. Visible evidence of urine leakage may be apparent on speculum examination of the vagina. Recurrent tumour or suspicious areas can be detected. Bimanual examination usually reveals at least a degree of pelvic thickening or induration. The bladder wall may be indurated and thickened. The vagina is often short, stenosed and indurated. There may be ulceration with necrotic slough. More severe generalised changes are the development of a "frozen" pelvis in which sheets of immobile fibrous tissue fix the pelvic structures and ensheath them. This mass of oedematous, thickened and fibrous pelvic tissue may be difficult to distinguish from tumour.

A fistula may be felt as well as seen. The margins are often indurated and inflamed. Where there is doubt about the presence of a vesico-vaginal fistula a three-swab test may be performed. This involves the presence of a urethral catheter in the bladder and three gauze swabs at different levels in the vagina. Blue dye (indigo-carmine or methylene blue) is introduced into the bladder and the swabs are checked for evidence of leakage. The worst possible situation is the presence of a compound fistula involving bowel and urinary tract associated with a small capacity bladder in a "frozen" pelvis.

The spectrum of our recent experience of urinary tract complications after pelvic radiotherapy is shown in the Appendix. In several of these patients more than one complication was present. It will be seen that radiation cystitis was the commonest complication but that both vesico-vaginal fistula and ureteric dilatation have been significant problems.

References

Albrecht KF (1981) Chirurgische problems nach strahlentherapie: Urologie. Langenbecks Arch Chir 355:199–204

Aldridge CW, Mason JT (1950) Ureteral obstruction in carcinoma of the cervix. Am J Obstet Gynecol 60:1272–1280

Altvater G, Imholz G (1960) Ureteral stenosis in carcinoma of the cervix uteri. Prognostic significance and surgical treatment. Geburtshilfe Frauenheilkd 20:1214–1229

Bloedorn FG, Young JD, Cuccia CA, Mercado R Jr, Wizenberg MH (1962) Radiotherapy in carcinoma of the bladder: possible complications and their prevention. Radiology 79:576–581

Boronow RC (1971) Management of radiation-induced vaginal fistulas. Am J Obstet Gynecol 110:1–8

Burns BC Jr, Everett HS, Brack CB (1960) Value of urologic study in the management of carcinoma of the cervix. Am J Obstet Gynecol 80:997–1004

Caldwell WL, Bagshaw MA, Caplan HS (1967) Efficacy of linear accelerator x-ray therapy in cancer of the bladder. J Urol 97:294–303

Chau PM, Fletcher GH, Rutledge FN, Dodd GD Jr (1962) Complications in high dose whole pelvic irradiation in female pelvic cancer. Am J Roentgenol Radium Ther Nucl Med 87:22–40

Cushing RM, Towell HM, Liegner LM (1968) Major urological complications following radium and x-ray therapy for carcinoma of the cervix. Am J Obstet Gynecol 101:750–755

Dean RJ, Lytton B (1978) Urological complications of pelvic radiation. J Urol 119:64–67

DeCosse JJ, Rhodes RS, Wentz WB, Reagan JW, Dworken HJ, Holden WD (1969) The natural history and management of radiation induced injury of the gastrointestinal tract. Ann Surg 170:369–384

Everett HS (1939) The effect of carcinoma of the cervix uteri and its treatment upon the urinary tract. Am J Obstet Gynecol 38:889–906

Everett HS, Brack CB, Farber GJ (1949) Further studies on the effect of irradiation therapy for carcinoma of the cervix upon the urinary tract. Am J Obstet Gynecol 58:908–923

Fowler JE Jr, Barzell W, Hilaris BS, Whitmoe WF Jr (1979) Complications of 125-iodine implantation and pelvic lymphadenectomy in treatment of prostatic cancer. J Urol 121:447–451

Friedman M, Lewis LG (1958) Irradiation of carcinoma of the bladder by a central intracavity radium or cobalt 60 source. (The Walter Reed technique). Am J Roentgenol 79:6–31

Golomb J, Waizbard E, Ienia A, Merimsky E (1986) Recurrent bladder perforation in chronic radiation cystitis. J Urol (Paris) 92:47–48

Graham JB, Abad RS (1967) Ureteral obstruction due to radiation. Am J Obstet Gynecol 99:409–415

Hiilesmaa VK, Vesterinen E, Nieminen U, Grohn P (1981) Carcinoma of the uterine cervix Stage III: a report of 311 cases. Gynaecol Oncol 12:99–106

Kaplan AL (1977) Post-radiation ureteral obstruction. Obstet Gynecol Survey 32:1–8

Kirchoff H (1960) Complication-abundant changes in the urinary tract after radiotherapy of cervical carcinoma. Geburtschilfe Frauenheilkd 20:34–39

Kjorstad KE, Martimbeau PW, Iversen T (1983) Stage 1B carcinoma of the cervix, the Norwegian Radium Hospital: results and complications. Gynecol Oncol 15:42–47

Kline JC, Buchler DA, Boone ML, Peckham BM, Carr WF (1972) The relationship of reactions to complications in the radiation therapy of cancer of the cervix. Radiology 105:413–416

Kottmeier HL (1964) Complications following radiation therapy in carcinoma of the cervix and their treatment. Am J Obstet Gynecol 88:854–866

Kottmeier HL, Gray MJ (1961) Rectal and bladder injuries in relation to radiation dosage in carcinoma of the cervix. Am J Obstet Gynecol 82:74–82

Lang EK, Wood M, Brown R et al. (1973) Complications in the urinary tract related to treatment of carcinoma of the cervix. South Med J 66:228–236

Lenz M, Cahill GF, Melicow MM, Donlan CP (1947) The treatment of cancer of the bladder by radium needles. Am J Roentgenol 58:486–492

Liegner LM, Taylor JA, Michaud NJ (1962) Super-voltage cobalt-60 treatment of bladder cancer: palliation or cure. J Urol 87:373–380

Lindholt J, Hansen PT (1986) Prostatic carcinoma: complications of megavoltage radiation therapy. Br J Urol 58:52–54

Lupton EW, Holden D, George NJR, Barnard RJ, Rickards D (1985) Pressure changes in the dilated upper urinary tract on perfusion at varying flow rates. Br J Urol 57:622–624

Miller LS, Crigler CM, Guinn GA (1964) Super-voltage irradiation for carcinoma of the urinary bladder. Radiology 82:778–785

Mollenkamp JS, Cooper JF, Kagan AR (1975) Clinical experience with super-voltage radiotherapy in carcinoma of the prostate: a preliminary report J Urol 113:374–377

Muram B, Oxorn H, Currie RJ, Drouin P, Walters JH (1981) Post-radiation ureteral obstruction: a reappraisal. Am J Obstet Gynecol 139:289–293

Nieminen U, Pollanen L (1970) Results of the treatment of carcinoma of the cervix uteri. Acta Obstet Gynecol Scand 49:321–325

O'Reilly PH, Shields RA, Testa HJ (1986) Nuclear medicine in urology and nephrology. Butterworths, London

Ram MD (1970) Visceral complications of super-voltage radiotherapy for carcinoma of the bladder. Br J Sur 57:409–412

Ray GR, Bagshaw MA (1975) The role of radiation therapy in the definitive treatment of adenocarcinoma of the prostate. Annu Rev Med 26:567–588

Ray GR, Cassady JR, Bagshaw MA (1973) Definitive radiation therapy of carcinoma of the prostate. Radiology 106:407–418

Riches E, Windeyer BW (1960) Modern trends in urology, 2nd series. Butterworths, London

Ruponen S (1977) Diagnostic and therapeutic aspects of cervical carcinoma based on the material of 991 cases. Acta Obstet Gynecol Scand (Supplement) 68

Sackett NB (1935) The prognosis of cancer of the cervix treated by irradiation. N Y State J Med 35:1153–1158

Schellhammer PF, El Mahdi AM (1983) Pelvic complications after definitive treatment of prostate cancer by interstitial or external beam irradiation. Urology 5:451–457

Schellhammer PF, Jordan GH, El Mahdi AM (1986) Pelvic complications after interstitial and external beam irradiation of urologic and gynecologic malignancy. World J Surg 10:259–268

Sewell RA, Braren V, Wilson SK, Rhamy RK (1975) Extended biopsy follow-up after full course radiation for resectable prostatic carcinoma. J Urol 113:371–373

Shingleton HM, Fowler WC Jr, Pepper ED Jr (1969) Ureteral strictures following therapy for carcinoma of the cervix. Cancer 24:77–83

Strockbine MF, Hancock JE, Fletcher GH (1970) Complications in 831 patients with squamous cell carcinoma of the intact uterine cervix treated with 3000 rads or more whole pelvis irradiation. Am J Roentgenol 108:293–304

Turner DPB (1961) Vesical haemorrhage after megavoltage irradiation. Br Med J 2:1462–1466

Twombly GH, Caceres E, Corscaden J (1952) The cause, incidence and treatment of irradiation injuries in the female pelvis. Am J Roentgenol 68:779–787

Unal A, Hamberger AD, Seski JC, Fletcher GH (1981) An analysis of the severe complications of irradition of carcinoma of the uterine cervix: treatment with intracavitary radium and parametrial irradiation. Int J Radiat Oncol Biol Phys 7:999–1004

Underwood PB, Lutz MH, Smoak DL (1977) Ureteral injury following irradiation therapy for carcinoma of the cervix. Obstet Gynecol 49:663–669

Villasanta U (1972) Complications of radiotherapy for carcinoma of the uterine cervix. Am J Obstet Gynecol 114:717–726

Whitaker RH (1979) The Whitaker test. Urol Clin N Am 6:529–539

Zerbig M, Teyssier P, Steg A (1983) Les sténoses urétérales après traitement des cancers du col utérin: fibrose post-radiothérapique ou récidive neoplasmique. J Chir (Paris) 120:503–513

8. Treatment of Radiation Urinary Tract Disease

R. J. Barnard and E. W. Lupton

Patients referred for the assessment of radiation disease of the urinary tract are those in whom the initial radiation reaction has subsided and urinary tract symptoms, with or without disorders of other pelvic organs, have appeared later (late disease). Rarely we see those in whom difficulties have arisen during treatment or in whom the initial reaction has never resolved (early disease).

The experience of many years has been intensified during the last five years when 300 patients with symptomatic urinary tract disease after radiotherapy have been assessed. Many had had carcinoma cervix for which treatment had been intensified in an attempt to improve survival. This applied particularly to the younger women in whom both the incidence and aggressiveness of the tumour had increased substantially in recent times.

General Principles

As with radiation bowel disease (RBD) the extent of the pathology is usually much greater than would be expected from a knowledge of the radiotherapy fields. This must be remembered when considering treatment of radiation urinary tract disease. In our experience the temporal sequence of events often shows a significant difference between the onset of urinary tract problems and RBD. The latter has in many instances appeared and been treated before the urinary tract symptoms appear. It is not clear whether this represents a greater resistance to damage by the tissues of the urinary tract or merely that this system is slower to react to that damage. However, several years ago, we began to assess the urinary tract in patients with RBD and it soon became apparent that evidence of damage could be demonstrated in the absence of symptoms. For this reason, we believe it is wise to assess the urinary tract of all patients with RBD so that early warning of future problems is available. It is also useful to have base-line information on renal function for future reference. Even subtle changes in overall or individual kidney function may well influence decisions about the timing and nature of operative intervention. In this context it would be helpful if renal form and function were evaluated in all cases before radiotherapy for pelvic malignancy. This is a counsel of perfection which, for various clinical and economic reasons, has not been achieved.

Since radiation changes are progressive, it is difficult to know at presentation whether further deterioration will occur with the passage of time. Apparently normal tissue may later develop ischaemic changes and jeopardise attempts at surgical repair. It is worthwhile noting that because the disease is basically due to ischaemia, any futher devascularisation by surgical intervention will add to the extent of damage. We must always be aware of the possibility of surgery for bowel disease accelerating the effects of ureteric and bladder radiation injury and vice versa.

The close anatomical relationship of the bowel with the urinary tract in the lower abdomen and pelvis together with the progressive ischaemic course of the disease process makes decisions about the nature and timing of surgery difficult. The choice between reconstruction and ablation and the determination of the optimal extent of resection are also difficult.

The overriding consideration in the management of urinary tract disease is preservation of renal function. This may be threatened by obstruction, infection or a combination of both. Ureters may be intrinsically strictured or extrinsically involved in the process of pelvic inflammation and progressive fibrosis. In practice the treatment of isolated involvement of ureters is rarely required and the combined management of ureteric and bladder problems is usually necessary.

Conservative Treatment

Symptoms associated with radiation urinary tract disease are usually confined to the lower urinary tract. Many patients experience an initial cystitis with symptoms similar to those of bladder infection, namely frequency, urgency, burning pain and varying degrees of haematuria. Indeed some may have a true urinary infection and appropriate antibiotic therapy may be required but in most instances urine cultures are sterile.

It is difficult to predict the natural history of radiation cystitis which persists for longer than one month after pelvic radiotherapy. Even when treatment is attempted, the condition may progress uninterrupted to extreme bladder fibrosis or fistula formation. Several forms of treatment have been advocated for radiation cystitis but nothing in our experience is uniformly successful. Many patients are reassured, following cystoscopy, by knowing that there is no evidence of tumour recurrence. They come to terms with their urinary frequency despite attempts at treatment being unsuccessful or in the absence of any treatment. Anticholinergic drugs give some relief in a small proportion of patients. Because the frequency is due to bladder inflammation and/or a low compliance bladder associated with wall fibrosis, one would not expect anticholinergic therapy to be as successful as in the treatment of functional disorders such as detrusor instability. Nevertheless it may be worth attempting to reduce urinary frequency by the use of propantheline, imipramine, terodiline or oxybutynin.

Pain associated with micturition can be helped by simple remedies such as alkalinisation of the urine and the use of Pyridium (phenazopyridine). In a few instances the intravesical instillation of dimethyl sulphoxide (Rimso) provides some relief (Shirley et al. 1978). In general, early irritative symptoms have abated with time and more persistent irritation has become better tolerated so that most patients have not required operative intervention.

Haematuria is a common problem and requires the usual investigation to exclude tumour as its cause. Once this has been done, haematuria which is infrequent and mild needs no active therapy. Haemorrhage can, however, pose serious problems due to its severity or repeated occurrence. Significant isolated episodes of haematuria in patients fit for anaesthesia should be managed cystoscopically and are considered later in this chapter. Repeated episodes may respond to intravesical chemical instillations. Alum (Ostroff and Chenault 1982; Kennedy et al. 1984) or formalin (Godec and Gleich 1983) may be used. Alum is less toxic than formalin and may be instilled without general anaesthetic. Formalin (1%–10%) instillation requires a general anaesthetic because it causes severe pain. Vesico-ureteric reflux must be excluded before its use and patients should be warned that it may well promote further bladder contraction. Recently, haemorrhage due to radiation cystitis has been successfully controlled by orally administered sodium pentosanpolysulphate (Parsons 1986).

Urinary incontinence sometimes causes problems. There are potentially several different reasons for urine leakage. Fibrous fixation of the sphincter mechanisms is not easily treated conservatively but pelvic floor exercises and perineal faradism may be worth trying. Catheters and collecting devices have a small role. We have seen one patient heal a vesico-vaginal fistula with an indwelling catheter inserted at a time when she was unfit for major surgery but this is a rare exception. Male incontinence devices such as condom urinals may be useful for sphincter problems after the treatment of carcinoma of prostate.

Pre-operative Preparation

Patients undergoing surgery for complications of radiotherapy are often anaemic and have poor nutritional status. Their routine investigations should include haematological and biochemical profiles, urine analysis and the usual general assessment of the cardiac and respiratory systems. Dehydration and electrolyte problems should be corrected by appropriate intravenous infusions. Severe anaemia may need pre-operative blood transfusion for its correction and parenteral nutrition may be required if there is metabolic depletion (see Chapter 6).

There may be significant renal impairment due to obstruction and/or infection. Obstructive uropathy can be relieved by the use of percutaneous nephrostomy under local anaesthetic as described in Chapter 3. When there is bilateral obstruction, fitness for anaesthesia can be achieved simply by inserting a nephrostomy tube on one side. If it is anticipated that prolonged resuscitation is required before corrective surgery it may be better to insert bilateral nephrostomies so as to protect both kidneys from the effects of obstruction. A percutaneous nephrostomy can be used to help predict functional recovery in an obstructed kidney. Percutaneous nephrostomies may also be valuable for the drainage of pyonephrosis associated with lower ureteric obstruction. It is often surprising how effectively pus drains through a fine calibre nephrostomy tube (7F). Larger percutaneous nephrostomy tubes with irrigating channels may also be useful. Dialysis may be necessary for severely ill patients with gross biochemical disturbance associated with renal failure. The renal impairment may be caused by obstruction or be due to acute tubular necrosis associated with septicaemia. Peritoneal dialysis is simpler to institute than haemodialysis but there may be problems with intra-abdominal sepsis and bowel adhesions. In our series, acute renal failure due to radiation disease has been much less common than renal failure due to recurrent tumour. Nevertheless, it should not be assumed, until proved, that tumour is the cause. We always alert the pathology department to the possible requirement for operative frozen sections which may be useful in decisions about the extent and nature of the operation.

The most significant problem in relation to post-radiation surgery is infection and most of our fatalities have been due to overwhelming septicaemia. For this reason, overt pre-operative infection is treated with appropriate antibiotics and all patients have operative cover with a broad-spectrum antibiotic such as cefuroxime, combined with metronidazole, which is continued well into the post-operative period.

In counselling patients pre-operatively, it is often difficult for the surgeon to give an accurate forecast of what procedures will be necessary. All eventualities need to be discussed including the possible requirement of stomas for the bowel and urinary tract. Even though bad for morale the possibility of recurrent or residual tumour needs to be discussed because operative procedures may need to be modified. It is helpful if a physiotherapist and a specialist stoma nurse can spend some time with the patient before the operation, explaining their roles in the management and giving some appropriate training in preparation for the post-operative period. We have found that stoma nurses are invaluable members of the team. They explain the procedures at length and help in selecting suitable sites for appropriate stomas. It may be reassuring for a patient to meet a selected former patient so that the practicalities of stoma management can be accurately demonstrated. Many patients find additional help from one of the descriptive booklets produced on stoma care.

Operative Treatment

Irradiated tissue heals less well than normal tissue and this should be uppermost in the surgeon's mind. It is not always possible to use abdominal incisions that will avoid previously irradiated areas and appropriate care in making and closing such incisions is necessary.

The presence of necrotic tissue in the pelvis is an invitation for infection and measures to remove all of this are necessary. In several of our patients this has necessitated a partial or complete pelvic clearance with appropriate conduit formation. Severely damaged areas of ureter or bladder should be adequately excised to improve the chances of healing in subsequent repairs.

Ureteric Disorders

The lower third of the ureter is inevitably exposed to radiation when pelvic tumours are treated. If there is ureteric damage, the usual initial finding is obstruction to one ureter only whether these patients are investigated as a result of ureteric symptoms, lower urinary tract symptoms or routinely in RBD. Obstruction of the contralateral ureter may develop sometime later and this possibility must be considered when deciding on the management of a single obstructed ureter.

In our series the obstruction has usually involved the lower third of the ureter but we have seen obstruction at or just below the pelvi-ureteric junction in three patients subsequent to pelvic irradiation. These cases have been successfully treated by standard pyeloplasty techniques. Histological examination of the removed segments has not offered a satisfactory explanation for the obstruction but it may be that this area of the ureter was rendered ischaemic when the distal vessels were affected by radiation endarteritis.

Once the site and length of a distal ureteric stricture has been established, its definitive management may be undertaken, provided that the residual function on the affected side is useful. In view of the possibility of contralateral ureteric obstruction at a later date, early intervention is not indicated for minor degrees of obstruction. We follow the patient by regular renography and operate if the situation deteriorates. For example, one of our patients with a ureteric stricture, impassable to even a guide wire, was followed by renography and showed no change in differential renal function over a period of 18 months. When eventually a slight fall-off in function was apparent she agreed to operative treatment.

We have temporised with ureteric dilatation using modern Lubriglide dilators when technically possible. This combined with an indwelling ureteric stent can allow time to observe the other ureter and, if renal function is equivocal, assess the recovery capability. Only on rare occasions in our patients has ureteric dilatation had a substantial long-term effect and this is the experience of other authors (Kaplan 1977). It should only be continued when the alternative is a nephrectomy.

Most established radiation ureteric strictures require surgical correction and the operative finding of intense peri-ureteric fibrosis explains the failure of more conservative methods of treatment. The type of surgery necessary is determined largely by the state of the lower urinary tract. Bladder fibrosis makes difficult the manipulation of that structure to facilitate reimplantation of the ureter. Boari flaps are not normally possible because of associated bladder disease. Only on one occasion have we managed to construct a satisfactory psoas hitch into which both ureters were implanted with a successful outcome (Fig. 8.1). All other ureteric strictures have been treated by interposing a segment of ileum or ileum/ caecum between the healthy ureter and the bladder and modifying the length of bowel substitute to increase the bladder capacity where this was reduced by fibrosis (Fig. 8.2.). The incorporation of the ileocaecal valve as an antireflux mechanism is attractive but needs careful consideration in the presence of RBD, as removal of the valve from the continuity of the intestinal tract may produce intractable diarrhoea.

When reimplanting the ureter into the bladder or anastomosing it to an intervening segment of bowel it is important to use healthy ureter above the radiation field. To avoid devascularisation gentle dissection is required for

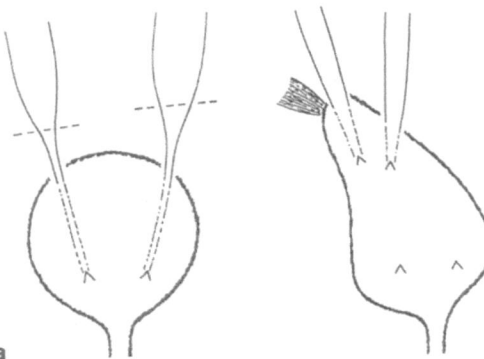

Fig. 8.1. Ureteric reimplantation and psoas hitch: **a** diagramatic representation: **b** IVU appearances 7 years later.

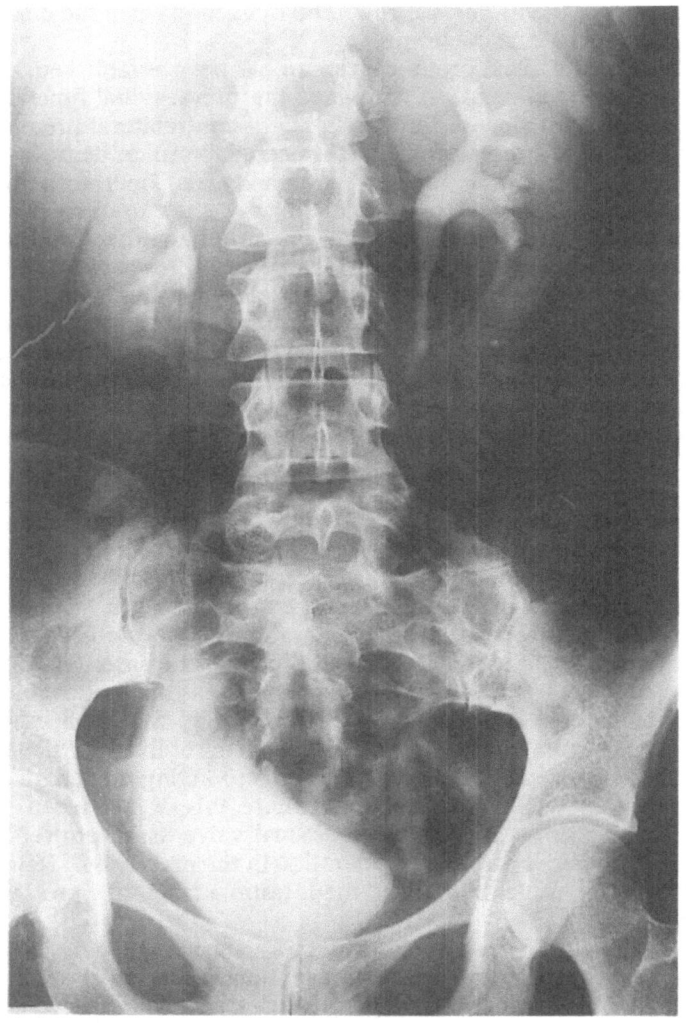

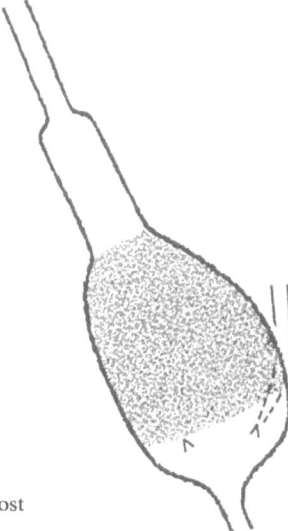

Fig. 8.2. Right uretero-ileo-caecocystoplasty for substitution of lost ureteric length and augmentation of bladder.

mobilisation of the ureter, the blood vessels should be included in the mobilised tissue and only the minimum length should be freed. For anastomosis of the ureter to interposed bowel we use the Wallace technique (1966). All ureteric anastomoses are stented with purpose-designed stents or 6/8F umbilical catheters which are left in position for approximately 10 days.

Ureteric fistula is much less common than stricture and we have only seen two in the past five years, one into the uterus and one into the vagina. In both of these cases it would seem likely that the primary tumour involved both structures and its destruction by radiotherapy allowed the fistula to develop. Once the diagnosis is established the operative treatment is the same as for ureteric stricture. It depends on the presence or absence of tumour and the extent of damage to the lower urinary tract.

Vesico-ureteric reflux has been reported in the literature (Albrecht 1981) but has not appeared as a clinical problem in our experience. If established by investigation the need for therapy will depend on the degree of interference, if any, with renal function and the severity of any symptoms. Should surgical treatment be necessary the general principles outlined above will apply.

Bladder Disease

The usual reasons for operative treatment in patients with urinary tract radiation disease are severe bladder changes. Although the operative procedure may improve upper urinary tract structure and function it is the lower tract symptoms that provide the main indication for surgery. Surgical procedures range from the simplest of endoscopic techniques to complex reconstructions or ablations of diseased pelvic tissue. The operative treatment of radiation bladder disease varies and depends on the severity of the disease and its symptoms.

Inflammation

If irritative symptoms become persistent and troublesome despite conservative treatment, cystoscopy may be appropriate to wash debris from the bladder and to assess the mucosal changes. Areas of slough and calcification can be resected transurethrally. This may provide symptomatic relief although slough tends to reform. There may be doubt about the presence of recurrent tumour in the bladder wall and biopsy may be indicated for this reason.

Haematuria

Cystoscopy is required for diagnostic purposes to exclude recurrent tumours as a cause of the bleeding. If radiation disease is demonstrated it is usually possible to locate the source of bleeding. The cystoscopy often shows multiple areas of telangiectasia, some of which start to bleed as a result of the examination itself. The bleeding areas are diathermised and it is desirable to "spot" diathermise the centre of each telangiectasis to prevent or delay any subsequent bleeding. This technique has rarely failed to halt the immediate problem but regular episodes of bleeding require more active treatment. It is at this stage the chemical instillation described previously may be indicated. Urgent cystoscopy may be required in some patients to relieve clot retention. If the haemorrhage proves intractable internal iliac artery embolisation can be successful. Rarely, urinary diversion, preferably combined with a simple cystectomy, is the only alternative.

Contracture

Diminished bladder capacity affects patients' lives to differing degrees and the requirement for active intervention is more likely in the "barrister" than the "gardener". In some patients the bladder capacity does improve without active treatment even when the bladder is believed to be irrevocably fibrosed. We have observed that some patients who refused surgery for small capacity bladders have coped for over 10 years and the condition has not significantly deteriorated.

Surgical attempts to increase the bladder capacity have involved several different techniques. Careful pre-operative assessment of the bladder is required to exclude new tumour formation by biopsy of any suspicious areas. In male patients, visual and if necessary urodynamic information about the bladder outlet is necessary; obvious obstruction should be corrected prior to cystoplasty. During the performance of cystoplasties for radiation disease care must be taken to use tissue that is healthy. The terminal ileum is often the site of some radiation damage which renders it inelastic and useless for cystoplasty. The sigmoid colon may be similarly damaged or the site of diverticular disease which makes it less useful.

Cystoplasty will require the use of significant lengths of bowel to achieve adequate bladder capacity and these may not be available where RBD is present. Attention must be paid to symptoms of RBD which may be worsened if a significant length of bowel is removed. Where bowel is used for replacing a damaged bladder or ureter it is essential that it has a good blood supply. Evidence included in Chapter 5 shows that vascular changes in the bowel may be much more extensive than the gross appearance indicates and this must be considered when selecting a length of bowel. Almost any accessible piece of bowel can be used for these operations and clearly which piece is used depends entirely on the prevailing anatomy and the degree of involvement of the intestine in the radiation disease.

Numerous types of cystoplasty are available in order to increase the bladder capacity in radiation disease. It is sometimes necessary to remove all of the diseased bladder and perform a substitution cystoplasty (Ong 1970; Turner-Warwick 1979; DeKlerk et al. 1979; Lilien and Camey 1984; Zinman and Libertino 1986; Goldwasser et al. 1987). It has been suggested that complete substitution is preferable to leaving any diseased bladder behind in radiation disease (Mundy 1986). It is our experience however that, if the bladder mucosa is not grossly abnormal, an augmentation cystoplasty will suffice. It may be better in cases with minimal trigonal disease to leave at least some of the bladder base for preservation of adequate vesical sensation (Kirby and Turner-Warwick 1987). Many methods of augmenting bladders have been described (Kuss 1959; Dounis et al. 1980; Bramble 1982; Kay and Straffon 1986). The bladder may be replaced or augmented using ileum, caecum or colon and discussions continue as to the relative merits of each of these patches (Goodwin 1987). For several years it has been suspected that reconstructed bladders using detubularised bowel are more satisfactory storage units than those using tubular intestinal segments. This has been supported by recent experimental work demonstrating that detubularised segments hold larger volumes before their wall tension rises (Concepcion et al. 1988). It has also been recognised that the modified bladder unit empties more efficiently if it is spherical rather than cylindrical (Chiang and Rosenfeld 1988; F. Shreiter, unpublished work presented at Urodynamic Society, Boston, USA, 4 June 1988).

In uncomplicated bladder fibrosis it has become our practice to perform a modified "clam" type of cystoplasty using at least 40–45 cm of detubularised bowel inserted in an "s" or "z" fashion (Fig. 8.3.). The actual portion of bowel has varied according to availability and in some instances we have had to be satisfied with less than optimal length. Rarely we have needed to use a cat's tail technique (Kirby and Turner-Warwick 1987) because of a short mesentery. In order to achieve satisfactory healing it is important that the "insert" has a good blood supply and the anastomosis is not under tension.

In the early post-operative period the bladder is drained by a wide bore (22–24F) plastic catheter to allow adequate drainage of mucus, debris and blood clot. The catheter is retained by either a small balloon or preferably by a nylon suture brought out through the bladder to the anterior abdominal wall. The abdomen and pelvis are generally drained by a single plastic catheter drain inserted through the anterior abdominal wall.

Fistula

We have seen vesico-vaginal fistula more often than complex fistula but in some cases a fistula has involved small bowel, bladder, vagina and large bowel with the production of an iatrogenic "cloaca". Vesico-vaginal fistula, as a single problem, occurs at varying times in relation to radiotherapy. Some appear during or soon after the treatment and are related to invasive necrotic tumours which slough and

a

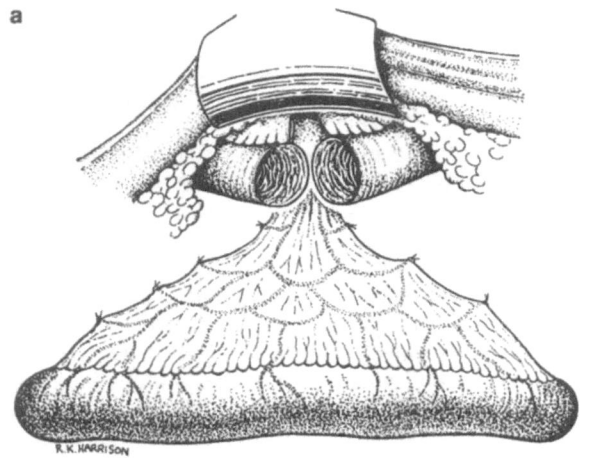

b

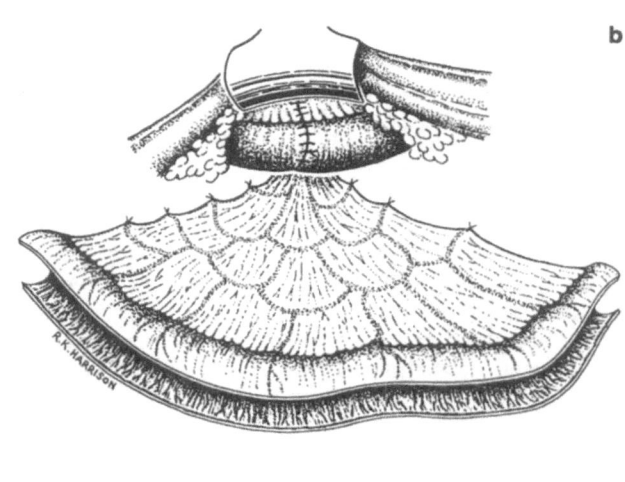

c

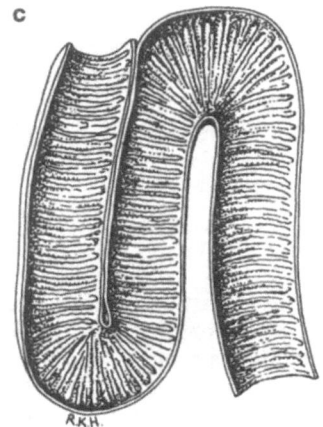

d

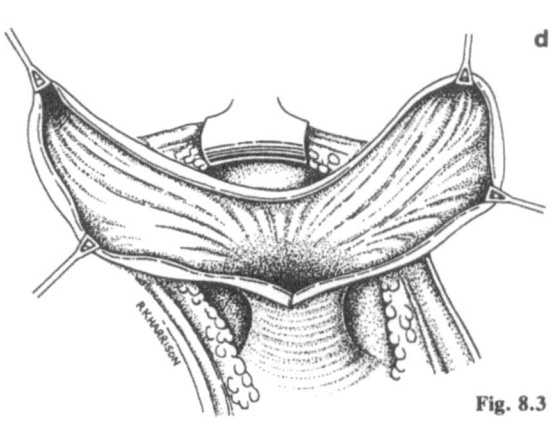

Fig. 8.3

Fig. 8.3. Augmentation of cystoplasty.
3a Loop of ileum isolated.
3b Isolated ileum divided along its anti-mesenteric border (detubularised).
3c Detubularised ileum sutured in S-shape (only one suture line shown).
3d Bladder remnant prepared for anastomosis of ileal augment.

leave the fistula. A fistula which occurs some time after therapy may be tumour-free and its management depends on clinical and histological examination of the area involved. Pure radiation fistula usually occurs within the first two years but can occur later.

If tumour is present in relation to the fistula the management is dependent on the surgical curability of the lesion. If operable, anterior pelvic clearance with urinary conduit formation is indicated. If inoperable, a simple urinary diversion will provide appropriate palliation. Some authorities have advocated that this should only be performed if life expectancy is in excess of six months (Lyndrup and Sorensen 1983). We feel that an individual decision has to be tailored to the patient so that a palliative procedure may be justified even for a short life-expectancy.

It is our practice to attempt a repair of the fistula when the patient has been shown to be tumour-free. At laparotomy, the initial assessment would include frozen section examination of any suspicious area. Care must be taken to avoid further injury to the blood supply of the preserved portion of the bladder. For small defects with minimal generalised bladder disease a γ-v-plasty of the posterior bladder wall (Fig. 8.4) together with closure of the vaginal defect and omental interposition may be suitable. As most of these patients have reduced bladder capacity, we have generally used an augmentation cystoplasty to replace the excised fistula and adjacent diseased bladder (Fig. 8.5). This is reinforced where possible with an omental covering. Boronow (1971) advocated the use of a labial fat pad on a pedicle as described by Martius (1929, 1956) (see Chapter 6). It is our view that, as laparotomy is necessary to assess the pelvis fully, it is usually easier to employ tissue derived from the abdomen.

Inevitably there may be some patients in whom most or all of the bladder will be removed in order to excise all the areas of necrosis. This may produce a

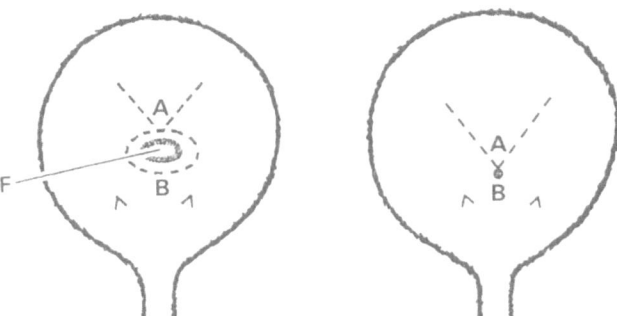

Fig. 8.4. Repair of vesico-vaginal fistula (F): Y-V plasty of posterior bladder wall, moving points A and B together after excision of fistula and surrounds.

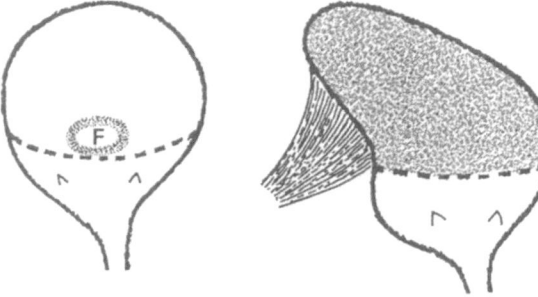

Fig. 8.5. Bladder reconstruction for contracture and vesico-vaginal fistula: excision of diseased bladder and augmentation cystoplasty using caecum.

situation where urinary diversion is necessary. Attempts can be made at reconstruction with a defunctioning urinary diversion (Fig. 8.6). The diversion can be closed at a later date but in practice patients may elect to keep their diversions rather than have further surgery.

A low fistula involving the urethra is treated by urinary diversion because we have found that the continence mechanisms are inevitably irreparably damaged. In contrast to the situation for cystoplasty, it is permissible to construct a conduit using bowel which has been mildly damaged by radiation, provided the ureters are healthy. Healing of uretero-conduit anastomoses has not been a problem.

Combined Urinary Tract and Bowel Problems

In facing the challenge of an ischaemic disease affecting potentially large segments of the bowel and urinary tract there is a need to be constantly aware of the effects of surgical treatment to one system affecting the structure and function of the other system. Surgery for isolated disease in the bowel may hasten the ischaemic changes in the urinary tract. Furthermore, by the time the urinary tract features present there may already have been large segments of radiation diseased bowel excised, leaving insufficient lengths for cystoplasty or ureteric

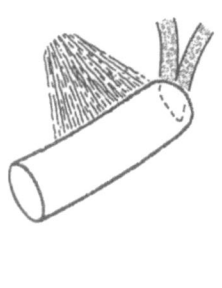 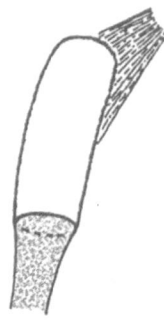

Fig. 8.6. Substitution cystoplasty using ileum (*right*) with temporary defunctioning ileal loop (*left*), which can be anastomosed to the cystoplasty at a later date.

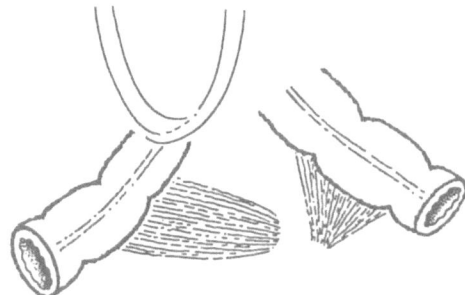

Fig. 8.7. Colon-loop diversion and end colostomy fashioned from adjacent segments of large bowel.

replacement. If there is sufficient bowel remaining, further reduction of intestinal length may produce problems such as malabsorption and diarrhoea. If the urinary tract is operated on first, the orientation of the mesentery of the bowel used for a cystoplasty may cause access problems during later bowel surgery.

Simultaneous surgery for diseased bowel and bladder are sometimes necessary. This provides the opportunity for healthy pieces of bowel proximal to radiation damaged segments to be used for urinary and genital tract reconstruction and/or urinary diversion (Schofield et al. 1989). This principle tends to minimise the number of required bowel anastomoses. For example, a piece of healthy small bowel proximal to an excised segment of radiation damaged small intestine can be used for bladder reconstruction. In the large bowel it may be possible to use two adjacent healthy proximal segments to fashion a colon loop diversion and an end-colostomy (Fig. 8.7). If the large bowel is used for cystoplasty there is the possibility of good antireflux ureterocolic anastomoses.

Complex fistulae involving bowel, bladder and vagina are difficult and individual problems which require careful evaluation and treatment. They represent extensive damage in the pelvis and many have required urinary and faecal diversion as the only feasible solution. Where there has been extensive necrosis and infection, diversion has been combined with radical ablation of the anterior and posterior pelvic contents. Less commonly it has proved possible to repair one or other of the excretory systems and divert the other. Exceptionally we have attempted to repair both. This inevitably involves the use of a temporary covering colostomy which is only closed if both systems are subsequently demonstrated to be intact.

It should be emphasised that, whatever the pathology associated with radiation disease, each operation is an individual event and it is not possible to give advice as to which procedure to use to cover all eventualities. It has largely been a matter of adapting established procedures to the individual situation.

Bladder Neck and Urethral Problems

Urethral Stricture

Stricture is not uncommon in male patients treated for prostatic or bladder carcinoma and generally occurs at the bladder outlet. The incidence of bladder neck and urethral fibrosis increases if radiotherapy has been administered immediately after a previous prostatic resection. For prophylaxis against this problem it is better to wait 4–6 weeks after resection before giving the radiotherapy (Schellhammer et al. 1986). Visual bladder neck incision or urethrotomy is usually effective for an established stricture but may have to be repeated on several occasions.

We have seen a radiation-induced urethral stricture in only one female patient. Dilatation and urethrotomy provided only short-lived relief and even when the lady was able to pass urine the continence mechanism was not fully effective. She required urinary diversion to control her symptoms.

Calcification

Calcification of necrotic tissue after pelvic radiation produces problems in the upper urethra. The areas can either be dislodged or resected with subsequent evacuation via the resectoscope. Over-aggressive resection or diathermy in the prostatic urethra must be avoided lest the resulting devascularisation produces a prostato-rectal fistula. The sloughing lesions in the proximal urethra take a long time to heal but repeated biopsy to exclude tumour recurrence is not usually necessary.

Incontinence

On occasions this has proved to be a post-irradiation problem in men treated for prostatic carcinoma extending into the distal sphincter. If it is a significant symptom, management has been by either an incontinence appliance or long-term catheterisation. Perhaps in the future the Brantley Scott artificial sphincter may be more liberally used in this situation (Scott 1978).

In the female where incontinence is more common such aids are not applicable. The cause of the problem is urethral and pelvic fibrosis impairing both intrinsic and extrinsic continence mechanisms. In our experience it has not proved possible to control the incontinence by Teflon injections (Politano et al. 1974) and the usual type of surgery employed for stress incontinence is not possible because of tissue fixation. Almost invariably, if there is significant leakage, a urinary diversion is necessary.

Urethral Fistula

There is a small but definite incidence of urethro-rectal fistula following the treatment of prostatic carcinoma. One of our patients developed a fistula between the urethra and the lower rectum several months after radiotherapy and a Hartmann's operation for rectal carcinoma. The fistula was exposed by a York Mason approach through the detubularised rectum (Mason 1972). The rectal muscle was used to cover the area of the defect. Post-radiation fistula involving the urethra in the female has been treated by urinary diversion.

Post-operative Care

Post-operative care follows the usual lines for major abdominal surgery. Nasogastric suction via a Ryles tube accompanied by intravenous infusion is continued until intestinal function shows signs of recovery. Antibiotic therapy is continued for up to 10 days depending upon progress and modified if necessary. Early mobilisation is usually possible and should be encouraged. Chest physiotherapy may well be necessary in older patients. Drains are usually removed on the fifth post-operative day and, dependent upon progress, bladder catheters are removed at 7–10 days. Theoretically, bladder emptying problems may occur after cystoplasty. We have found that this is rarely a problem after treating radiation disease. If it does occur the patients may be taught clean intermittent self-catheterisation (Lapides et al. 1972). Moral support during a sometimes difficult post-operative period is vital. Psychiatric help may occasionally be required.

Complications

Many of the surgical procedures for radiation urinary tract disease are major operations. The patients are therefore potentially subject to the usual problems after major abdominal or pelvic surgery. Particularly important are the risks of infection and anastomotic leakage. If healthy tissue has been used, bowel anastomoses should not break down. Continued urine leakage from the reconstructed bladder or ureter may be a problem but the liberal use of the omentum and appropriate splintage and catheter drainage will minimise the incidence. If urine leakage is becoming troublesome, it may be expedient to insert percutaneous nephrostomy tubes until healing of anastomoses has occurred or the patient is well enough for further surgery. Urine leakage from the ureteroconduit anastomosis following urinary diversion may be helped simply by placing a catheter through the stoma into the conduit.

Sepsis is a constant threat with these patients. It is best avoided by a wide excision of necrotic pelvic tissue and good antibiotic cover. Unexplained pyrexia requires early assessment with blood cultures and alteration of the antibiotic regime as necessary. Nevertheless, failure to control sepsis leading to septicaemia has been the greatest cause of early post-operative morbidity and mortality.

Incontinence may occur for a variety of reasons after cystoplasty (Webster and Goldwasser 1987). The use of detubularised bowel minimises the tendency to "unstable" contractions in the bowel patch. Troublesome contractions may be treated with anticholinergic therapy or drugs which inhibit intestinal motility, for example diphenoxylate hydrochloride (Lomotil). Outlet obstruction in male subjects is corrected by the appropriate transurethral procedure. Intermittent self-catheterisation may be necessary for persistently large residual urines in both sexes but, as previously stated, emptying difficulties have been uncommon in this group of patients.

Only rarely in our experience has late fibrotic change been a problem. Recurrent ureteric strictures are uncommon. Indeed, the major late complications of surgery for radiation disease, such as fistula formation, are most likely to occur when unrelated surgery affects contiguous structures. A typical example was seen when one of our patients developed a vesico-vaginal fistula shortly after an aortic bifurcation graft but many years after her original radiotherapy.

Prognosis

There has been a dearth of reports on the long-term prognosis of radiation disease of the urinary tract. In our own initial series of 62 patients (see Appendix) 22 patients had died by the time of the 3-year assessment. The main cause of death was recurrent tumour but it is noticeable that overwhelming sepsis was a prominent feature. The combination of severe bowel and urinary tract disease produces a higher risk of life-threatening septicaemia. It is gratifying that amongst those patients who remain alive a high proportion are well and symptom-free.

References

Albrecht KF (1981) Chirurgische problems nach strahlentherapie: Urologie. Langenbecks Arch Chir 355:199–204

Boronow RC (1971) Management of radiation-induced vaginal fistulas. Am J Obstet Gynecol 110:1–8

Bramble FJ (1982) The treatment of adult enuresis and urge incontinence by entero-cystoplasty. Br J Urol 54:693–696

Chiang H, Rosenfeld RE (1988) The "s" shaped detubularised ileo-cystoplasty for bladder augmentation. J Urol 139:145a

Concepcion RS, Koch MO, McDougal S, Richards WO (1988) Detubularised intestinal segments in urinary tract reconstruction: why do they work? J Urol 139:310a

DeKlerk JN, Lambrechts W, Biljoen I (1979) The bowel as substitute for the bladder. J Urol 121:22–24

Dounis A, Abel DJ, Gow JG (1980) Caeco-cystoplasty for bladder augmentation. J Urol 123:164–167

Godec CJ, Gleich P (1983) Intractable hematuria and formalin. J Urol 130:688–691

Goldwasser B, Barrett DM, Benson RC Jr (1987) Complete bladder replacement using the detubularised right colon. In: King LR, Stone AR, Webster GD (eds) Bladder reconstruction and continent urinary diversion. Year Book Medical Publishers Inc, Chicago London, pp 360–366

Goodwin WE (1987) Experiences with intestine as a substitute for the urinary tract. In: King LR, Stone AR, Webster GD (eds) Bladder reconstruction and continent urinary diversion. Year Book Medical Publishers Inc, Chicago London, pp 9–29

Kaplan AL (1977) Post-radiation ureteral obstruction. Obstet Gynecol Surv 32:1–8

Kay R, Straffon R (1986) Augmentation cystoplasty. Urol Clin N Am 13:295–306

Kennedy C, Snell ME, Witherow RO (1984) Use of alum to control intractable vesical haemorrhage. Br J Urol 56:673–675

Kirby RS, Turner-Warwick R (1987) Substitution cystoplasty. In: King LR, Stone AR, Webster GD (eds) Bladder reconstruction and continent urinary diversion. Year Book Medical Publishers Inc. Chicago London, pp 41–63

Kuss R (1959) Colocystoplasty rather than ileo-cystoplasty. J Urol 82:587–589

Lapides J, Diokno AC, Silber SJ (1972) Clean intermittent self-catheterisation in the treatment of urinary tract disease. J Urol 107:458–461

Lilien OM, Camey M (1984) 25-year experience with replacement of the human bladder (Camey procedure). J Urol 132:886–891

Lyndrup J, Sorensen BL (1983) Palliative urinary conduit diversion in cases of intolerable urinary discomfort. Gynecol Oncol 16:360–364

Martius H (1929) Sphincter und Harnröhrenplastik aus dem M. bulbocavernosus. Chirurgie 17:49

Martius H (1956) In: McCall ML, Bolten KA (eds) Operative gynecology. Little, Brown and Company, Boston

Mason AY (1972) Trans sphincteric exposure of the rectum. Ann R Coll Surg Engl 51:320–331

Mundy AR (1986) Cystoplasty. In: Mundy AR (ed) Current operative surgery: urology. Ballière Tindall, Eastbourne, pp 140–159

Ong GB (1970) Colocystoplasty for bladder carcinoma after radical total cystectomy. Ann R Coll Surg Engl 46:320–336

Ostroff EB, Chenault OW Jr (1982) Alum irrigation for the control of massive bladder haemorrhage. J Urol 128:929–930

Parsons CL (1986) Successful management of radiation cystitis with sodium pentosanpolysulfate. J Urol 136:813–814

Politano VA, Small MP, Harper JM, Lynne CM (1974) Peri-urethral teflon injection for urinary incontinence. J Urol 111:180–183

Schellhammer PF, Jordan GH, El Mahdi AM (1986) Pelvic complications after insterstitial and external beam irradiation or urologic and gynecologic malignancy. World J Surg 10:259–268

Schofield PF, Barnard RJ, Tindall VR (1989) Surgical treatment of carcinoma involving the vagina. Br J Surg 76:816–817

Scott FB (1978) The artificial sphincter in the management of incontinence in the male. Urol Clin N Am 5:375–391

Shirley SW, Stewart BH, Mirelman S (1978) Dimethyl sulfoxide in treatment of inflammatory genitourinary disorders. Urology 11:215–220

Turner-Warwick R (1979) Cystoplasty. Urol Clin N Am 6:259–264

Wallace DM (1966) Ureteric diversion using a conduit: a simplified technique. Br J Urol 38:522–527

Webster GD, Goldwasser B (1987) Management of incontinence after cystoplasty. In: King LR, Stone AR, Webster GD (eds). Bladder reconstruction and continent urinary diversion. Year Book Medical Publishers Inc. Chicago London, pp 75–86

Zinman L, Libertino JA (1986) Right colocystoplasty for bladder replacement. Urol Clin N Am 13:321–331

9. Conclusions and the Future

P. F. Schofield and E. W. Lupton

Bowel and urinary tract symptoms which occur during and shortly after therapeutic radiation are well known and the corresponding histopathology is becoming clearer but the relationship to late radiation change is still obscure. This later reaction produces vascular damage and fibrosis leading to ischaemic changes. It is these later changes which in some patients may lead to severe clinical problems in both the intestine and the urinary tract.

It is apparent that effort should be made to reduce the incidence of these changes. The techniques of radiotherapy are well established but these therapeutic regimes run in a narrow therapeutic range in order to maximise cancer control but minimise unacceptable morbidity. The radiotherapist should recognise those patients who are in a higher risk category for radiation disease and tailor the treatment regimes accordingly. In addition, the higher risk of radiation carried out *after* an operation should be recognised. This may be ameliorated not only by alteration of the radiotherapy regime but by the surgeon realising the heightened risk and using some pelvic exclusion procedure. The possibility of cyto-protection by either systemic or intraluminal agents during the course of radiotherapy has been little explored but offers some hope for a reduction in the incidence of radiotherapy injury to normal tissues in the future.

Recent unexpected rises in morbidity rates with increases in the incidence of disorders of the bowel and urinary tract due to radiation change have been reported in many different centres. Despite this, the incidence of pelvic radiation disease is low across the population of Western Europe and the USA compared with that of inflammatory disease of the bowel and urinary tract. Since pelvic radiation disease is a rare phenomenon in the routine practice of coloproctology and urology, such a diagnosis is less likely to be considered in a practice which deals infrequently with the problem. Furthermore, there is considerable temptation to attribute abdominal and pelvic symptoms after radiotherapy for cancer to the presence of residual or recurrent tumour. Clinical awareness of the possible diagnosis of pelvic radiation disease is paramount. It is true that radiation disease and tumour recurrence can co-exist but it is all too easy to dismiss a complex problem as incurable when no tumour is present.

Awareness of the possible diagnosis needs to be matched with a willingness to thoroughly investigate these cases. It may be difficult to completely appraise the problems of a severely ill patient so that all factors contributing to the severity of the radiation disease are known before the planning of extensive surgery. To this end we have found that a multidisciplinary approach to management is highly advantageous. The early involvement of a coloproctologist and a urologist in the combined clinical assessment is valuable and the availability of dedicated radiological expertise is most useful.

All radiotherapy in the North West of England is carried out in one centre which serves a population in excess of five million people. This central arrangement for the treatment of pelvic tumours has provided a large study population from a wide geographical area and has given us an unusual experience of the associated problems. The experience of dealing with several hundred patients suffering from pelvic radiation disease has helped us to decide on coherent treatment policies and in particular has taught us when not to operate.

The fact that the main pathological sequelae of radiation damage are ischaemic has important implications for therapy. Minor injury may resolve completely in both the bowel and the urinary tract. Moderate injury will produce repair processes which will inevitably result in fibrosis of the involved organs. This will lead to strictures in cylindrical viscera such as the ureter and bowel which frequently require surgical correction. In a spherical organ such as the bladder, fibrosis will produce diminished capacity. It may be possible to live with the resulting symptoms but reconstructive augmentation may become necessary.

More severe damage will produce emergency situations such as peritonitis and compound fistulae. Because of the life-threatening nature of these problems, the timing of surgical intervention for the whole spectrum of damage is difficult. Since the disease is due to *progressive* ischaemia, early surgery may be followed by further radiation-induced problems. On the other hand, delay may lead to severe illness from metabolic depletion or septicaemia. Reconstructive procedures are not as easy as in the non-irradiated pelvis and even impeccably constituted anastomoses may break down because of imperfect healing if poorly vascularised tissue is used. The extent of the radiation change may be greater than is suspected from naked eye examination of the abdominal and pelvic contents. This applies particularly to the small and large bowel where healing of anastomoses may be compromised by excision of too short a segment of bowel. Another reason for a radical approach when committed to surgery is the need to remove potentially infected tissue. Residual bacteria in ischaemic tissue will produce persistent foci of infection with tissue destruction and the risk of life-threatening septicaemia. Wide excision of diseased tissue with good broad-spectrum antibiotic cover is mandatory. There is little or no place for diverting procedures alone as this does not allow sepsis to resolve.

After radical resection the salvage procedures should be reconstructive, if possible. It is preferable to augment or replace a bladder rather than opt for a permanent urinary diversion and to perform a colo-anal anastomosis rather than an abdomino-perineal excision of the rectum, if this can be done safely. The use of well-vascularised tissue for reconstruction is an easily understood principle. In practice the distal anastomosis line often proves problematical. This applies equally to the bladder and to the large bowel. The distal portions are fixed in position and lie in the maximally irradiated areas. Restorative procedures may have to be abandoned in favour of resection with a permanent urostomy or colostomy, on occasions. Where possible the liberal use of omentum or labial flaps will aid the healing properties of these low anastomoses.

The multidisciplinary approach to surgical treatment has enabled the use of well-vascularised colon for simultaneous reconstruction of the diseased urinary or genital tract after excision of radiation-damaged bowel. Normal colon can be used to replace a diseased vagina, to act as a urinary conduit or for augmentation of the bladder. It is preferable to use a piece of large bowel adjacent to resected colon for urinary or genital reconstruction rather than a separate segment of small bowel. The number of suture lines and hence the risk of anastomotic leakage is minimised. Such patients often have poor tissues as a result of the general effects of infection and the hypercatabolic process. Anastomotic leakage on top of these already existing difficulties is usually disastrous.

Not only is surgical technique important but good pre-operative and post-operative care will improve the results of surgery. We would mention the great importance of the highly skilled nursing care that these patients must receive. Accurate observation and attention to many details are vital to success. Support of these ill patients includes aspects such as total parenteral nutrition and antibiotics but psychological support from a team which is expert in management of these problems is invaluable.

It should always be remembered that pelvic radiation disease is potentially progressive. As illustrated in the appendix, we have seen cases presenting 20 years after treatment. Urinary tract disease is less likely to produce troublesome symptoms than bowel disease. However, there is a real risk of undetected renal functional impairment due to insidious ureteric stricturing. There is a case for the indefinite follow up of irradiated patients even after the risks of tumour recurrence have faded. Such an approach may not be logistically possible in a busy clinical situation. Nevertheless, our own practice is to follow patients with bowel disease carefully to ensure that they are not developing urinary tract disease and vice versa.

In summary we would emphasise the following points as being the most important principles of management of pelvic radiation disease:

1. Clinical awareness of the diagnosis even many years after the radiotherapy.
2. A multidisciplinary approach to management.
3. Conservative treatment for as long as possible.
4. When surgery is required, be radical with the excision of diseased tissue.
5. Use reconstruction when it is safe but consider a covering proximal diversion of the urinary stream or faeces.
6. As a last resort use ablative salvage procedures such as cystectomy and urinary diversion, nephrectomy or abdomino-perineal excision of the rectum with colostomy.

Even in the best hands, attempts to cure cancer by radiotherapy will inevitably result in a small incidence of these problems. Surgeons must aspire to increasingly sophisticated and more clinically acceptable methods of reconstruction. The problems in the bladder and rectum are similar in that we wish to produce an adequate reservoir with a satisfactory controlling sphincter. Bladder augmentation and colonic pouches have begun to address the reservoir question. The sphincter mechanism is still an unresolved problem when significant radiation disease affects these areas. With the evolution of devices such as artificial sphincters we can look to further improvement in the quality of life for patients suffering from this interesting and challenging disorder.

Appendix

This appendix contains detailed information on the investigations, treatment and outcome of patients with radiation disease. It is mainly based on patients seen in the late 1970s and early 1980s in whom we have knowledge of the longer term outcome.

We have analysed 100 consecutive patients with bowel disease and 62 successive patients with urinary tract disease. Also included are details of radiological investigation in 70 patients with bowel and/or urinary tract disease.

Our recent experience of radiation problems is shown in the final table which contains 100 patients treated in 1987–88.

Table A.1. Bowel disease at presentation (site) (*n*=100)

Colon or rectum	66
Ileum	19
Both	15

Table A.2. Colostomy alone – reviewed 1959; outcome at 5 years (*n*=18)

	Dead		Alive
Operative	2		
Urinary tract disease	3		
Septicaemia	4		
Recurrent tumour	5		
Total	14	*Total*	4

Table A.3. Ileal resection (1977–1982); outcome at 5 years ($n=33$)

	Dead		Alive
Operative	0	Urinary tract disease	6
Urinary tract disease	4	Further bowel disease	2
Recurrence	6	Well	15
Total	10	*Total*	23

Table A.4. Colonic resection (1977–1982); outcome at 5 years ($n=56$)

Restorative resection ($n=37$)				Abdomino-perineal ($n=19$)			
	Dead		Alive		Dead		Alive
Operative	2	Urinary tract disease	6	Operative	0	Further urinary tract disease	4
Urinary tract disease	4	Further bowel disease	4	Urinary tract disease	3	Further bowel disease	1
Recurrence	5	Well	16	Recurrence	3	Well	8
Total	11	*Total*	26	*Total*	6	*Total*	13

Table A.5. Renography – before definitive treatment
(48 patients – 96 kidneys)

Function		
Normal		75
Unilateral	non-function	3
	poor (20%)	7
	impaired (20–40%)	7
Bilateral	poor/impaired	4
Excretion		
Normal		48
Obstructed		15
Non-obstructive delay		8
Equivocal		3
Slow (no frusemide)		11
Poor/non-function		11

Table A.6.   Cystoscopy findings in 60 patients

Radiation cystitis	
Mild/moderate	32
Severe	13
Fistula	
Vesico-vaginal	12
Recto-vesico-vaginal	6
Vesico-colic	1
Vesico-vagino-colic	1
Vesico-perineal	2

Table A.7.   Urinary tract disease: final diagnosis in 62 patients (more than one pathology in 33 cases)

Radiation cystitis	45
Vesico-vaginal fistula	12
Unilateral ureteric obstruction	10
Bilateral ureteric obstruction	8
Non-obstructive/unspecified dilatation	10
Recto-vesico-vaginal fistula	5
Other fistulae	5

Table A.8.·   Urinary tract disease: surgical procedures (40 in 35 patients)

Ileal/colon loop diversion	20
Bladder reconstruction	9
Pelvic clearance	3
Ureteric reimplantation	2
Ureteric dilatation	3
Other	3

Table A.9.   Outcome in urinary tract disease (n=62)

Dead		Alive	
Post-operative	4	"Cystitis"	9
Septicaemia	6	Pelvic/loin pain	3
Renal failure	1	Other symptoms	3
Unrelated	1	Well	25
Recurrent tumour	10		
Total	22	*Total*	40

Table A.10. Distribution of radiological abnormalities

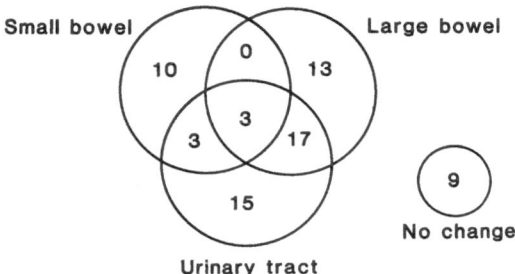

Table A.11. Radiology: small bowel

Patient no.	Abnormal plain films	Abnormal barium studies							Time from XRT
		Mucosa		Calibre		Wall		Fistula	
		Smooth	Irregular	Stenotic	Dilated	Thickening	Fixity		
4							+		3
6	+								1
31					+			+	5
33			+			+	+		1
37	+								6/12
38[a]			+	+	+	+			5/12
38[b]	+								2
41	+								2/12
43	+					'			1
45	+								5/12
46		+		+	+	+			1/12
47	+								2/52
48	+								9/12
50								+	1/12
55	+								1
59	+								3
63			+			+	+		2

[a] 1st examination.
[b] 2nd examination.

Table A.12. Radiology: large bowel

Patient no.	Length (cm)	Stricture						Fistula	Wide pre-sacral space	Time	Comment
		Site			Mucosa						
		Recto-sigmoid	Mid sigmoid	Prox. sigmoid	Smooth	Irregular	Normal				
1	4		+		+					10/12	
2			+							2	Complete obstruction
3								+		2	Fistula to abscess cavity
4	20			+		+				1	
7						+				1	Mucosal ulceration. No stricture
11	12		+		+					2	Angulation
15	10					+		+		9/12	Recto-jejunal
16	14	+			+					1	
17	8	+			+					1	
20	10	+			+					1	
21								+			Recto-vaginal
24	15								+	1	
27	10				+					1	
29								+		2	Recto-vaginal (+vesico-vaginal)
33	10[a]	+			+				+	1	Progressive narrowing & lengthening of stricture over 12/12
	20[b]	+				+			+	1	
35	8		+			+				9/12	
36	20		+						+	20	
37	10	+				+				2	Two separate strictures
	8		+		+						
40	7		+		+					5	
42	3		+			+				1	
44	4	+							+	1	Two separate strictures
	11		+								
51	5		+		+					8/12	
52	20		+		+				+	7/12	
56	20		+			+				1	
57	7		+							2	Prox. muscle hypertrophy
58			+							1	Stricture but poor Ba. coating – not fully assessable
61	9			+		+				1	"Stricture in stenosis"
64	13	+				+				7/12	
65		+							+	1	Two separate strictures
			+							1	
66	7		+			+				10/12	"Stricture in stenosis"
67	6		+			+				8/12	
68	15	+			+					7	Now progressive over 4 years
70	28		+							14	

[a] 1st examination.
[a] 2nd examination.

Table A.13. Radiology: Urinary tract

Patient no.	Ureter				Bladder					Time
	Right		Left		Size	Shape	Thickening	Mucosa irregular	Fistula[a]	
	Obstructed	Stricture (cm)	Obstructed	Stricture (cm)						
3				4						10/12
4	+	2	+	2			+			1
5	+						+			6/12
6	+		+	1.5		+	+			1
7			+	8b	+			+		1
8			+						RVVF	1
9			+	+						2
10	+		+	2						5/12
11			+							1
12	+	2	+					+	VVF	1
13					+		+	+		2
17	+	2	+	5					VVF	1
20	+	2	+	2		+	+			1
21	+	2							VVF	1
22	+		+	4						3
24	+	2					+			1
25	+	5							VVF	1
26	+	4				+	+	+		1
27	+	2	+	3						1
28	+	1								1
29	+		+	4					RVVF	1
31	+	5	+						VVF	3
32	+	2	+	2						1
33			+	8						3
34	+	3						+	VVF	1
35	+		+						UCF	9/12
37					+		+	+		1
39	+		+	2b	+		+		VVF	1
42	+	3	+	6b		+	+			1
48	+	4b								8/12
51					+		+	+		9/12
52	+						+	+		3
53	+	6	+	6			+	+		2
56	+	2	+	2	+		+			2
58								+		1
66	+	5	+		+				VVF	10/12
68	+	6	+	3		+	+	+		10
69	+								VVF	1

[a] RVVF, recto-vaginal-vesical fistula; VVF, vesico-vaginal fistula; UVF, uretero-vaginal fistula; UCF, uretero-colic fistula.
[b] High stricture.

Table A14. Pelvic radiation disease 1987–1989 (n=100)

Site primary tumour	Type of radiation	No. of patients	Site of disease		Bowel and urinary tract	No. of operations	
			Bowel	Urinary tract		Bowel	Urinary tract
Uterus	Ext. beam+intracavitary	56	26	9	21	33	18
	Intracavitary only	20	8	8	4	8	9
Prostate	Ext. beam	15	15	–	–	6	–
Bladder	Ext. beam	9	9	–	–	4	–

Subject Index